Don't Let Them Die

HIV/AIDS, TB, Malaria and the Healthcare Crisis in Africa

Published by
Adonis & Abbey Publishers Ltd
P.O. Box 43418
London
SE11 4XZ
http://www.adonis-abbey.com

First Edition, February 2006

Copyright © Chinua Akukwe

British Library Cataloguing-in-Publication Data

A catalogue record for this book is available from the British
Library

ISBN 1-905068-24-7

Cover Design MegaGraphix

Printed and bound in Great Britain

Don't Let Them Die

HIV/AIDS, Malaria, Tuberculosis and the Healthcare Crisis in Africa

By Chinua Akukwe

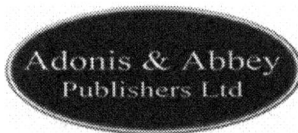

Adonis & Abbey
Publishers Ltd

Dedication

This book is dedicated to two set of critical players in the HIV/AIDS, TB and Malaria remedial efforts in Africa:

First, print and electronic media journalists and editors in Africa and around the world who, against popular opinion and political expediency, decided to focus on the devastating impact of HIV/AIDS, TB and Malaria in Africa. These journalists, especially those in Africa, were the first to give me the opportunity to write on HIV/AIDS and to push ideas that were not widely acceptable when I became actively involved in HIV/AIDS remedial efforts. I will continue to owe these journalists a great debt of gratitude.

Second, Africa's frontline health workers. These workers continue to perform miracles in various health institutions across the continent. These health workers work under trying circumstances in congested urban clinics, dilapidated primary health care centers and dispensaries in rural areas and crowded missionary institutions in Africa. These health workers, perhaps, have suffered more than most people involved in the remedial efforts against HIV/AIDS, TB and Malaria, since they are unable to provide timely care to their patients due to lack of medicines, proper infrastructure and financial support. The frontline health workers are the first line of defense against HIV/AIDS, TB and Malaria. Yet, these frontline health workers are often forgotten in the design, implementation, monitoring and evaluation of health programs and services in Africa.

Acknowledgement

I thank Jideofor Adibe and his editors at the Adonis & Abbey Publishers, London, United Kingdom, for their wonderful job of making this book a reality. Jideofor Adibe provided wide counsel, tactful encouragement and availed me of his comprehensive knowledge of the publishing industry regarding choice of materials for this book, the arrangement and other logistics.

I am very grateful to George Nubo, the editor in chief of the THE PERSPECTIVE magazine, based in Atlanta, United States. George Nubo provided an important platform for me to share my views on HIV/AIDS, TB and Malaria from my earliest days of involvement in HIV/AIDS remedial efforts.

I am also grateful to Terri Schure and Shane Tasker, the editor-in-chief/founder and the web-editor, respectively, of the WORLDPRESS.ORG, one of the most influential web portals, today. As a contributing editor, I had unique opportunities to reach a wider audience and to benefit from the excellent articles posted by other authors in WORLDPRESS.ORG.

I remain appreciative of the disposition of Chuck Odili, the publisher of NIGERIAWORLD.COM, an early supporter and promoter of my writings on healthcare issues in Africa.

I thank, Chuks Iloegbunam, one of Nigeria's most celebrated journalists and a columnist for the Vanguard Newspapers in Nigeria for his encouragement and support. Chuks Iloegbunam helped me sharpen my thinking on HIV/AIDAS, TB and Malaria, and, advised me on how to communicate my ideas to a wider audience.

I thank the editors of all journals, newspapers, web portals, radio and television programs in the United States, Africa and other parts of the world who allowed me to articulate my view on HIV/AIDS, TB and Malaria remedial efforts through their medium of communication.

I thank former US Congressman Ronald V. Dellums for his remarkable foresight and leadership of HIV/AIDS remedial efforts in Africa. I benefited immensely from his leadership and commitment as a member of the Board of Directors of the Constituency for Africa (CFA) which he served as the Chairman.

I also benefited from the passionate commitment to international development efforts in Africa from former US Congressman, former US Secretary of Urban and Housing Development and former Republican Vice-Presidential Candidate, Jack Kemp. As the Vice Chairman of CFA, Jack Kemp brought a unique, can-do insight of a top policy maker with experience in both the private and public sector.

I thank the Secretary-General of the United Nations, Kofi Annan for his extraordinary leadership on HIV/AIDS issues in Africa and throughout the world. Honorable Kofi Annan skillfully utilized the stature of his high office and his firm convictions to mainstream HIV/AIDS and other health issues in UN operations. The Secretary-General's contributions in mobilizing global support against HIV/AIDS will be a lasting testament of his tenure as the head of the UN.

I thank my fellow board of directors of the Constituency for Africa for their work on behalf of Africa. I also thank my colleagues at the George Washington University School of Public Health and the GWU Africa Center for Health and Security for their encouragement and support. GWU Provost, John Williams, Ms. Kristen Krapf-Campbell and Leroy Charles of the Africa Center have been major supporters of my work.

Finally, I thank my friends and mentors, Melvin Foote, Sidi Jammeh, Mohammad Akhter, George Haley, Elaine Murphy, late Honorable Olikoye Ransome-Kuti and late P.I. Okolo for their wise counsel and support throughout the years.

Table of Contents

PART V: AIDS IN AFRICA AND THE RESPONSIBILITY OF THE WEST

FOREWORD

When Chinua Akukwe was the Vice Chairman of the Executive Committee and Governing Board of the National Council for International Health (NCIH) now known as the Global Health Council, Washington, DC, he invited me to an international semi-nar series he convened and moderated in Washington, DC. In my presentation on HIV/AIDS in Africa, I challenged Dr. Akukwe and other Africans living and working in the West to join the then nascent effort to fight the AIDS epidemic in Africa. I specifically challenged all Africans in top positions in the academia, research organizations, the public sector, the private sector and the civil society to commit their time and resources to AIDS remedial efforts in Africa.

I am glad that Chinua Akukwe answered the call. Dr. Akukwe not only answered the call but also agreed to join the board of directors of the Constituency for Africa (CFA), Washington, DC which I serve as the Chief Executive Officer. Today, Chinua Akukwe is well known for his work on Africa's health and development issues.

This book is a lasting testament to Dr. Akukwe's significant contributions to AIDS remedial efforts in particular and healthcare in general, in Africa. This book is also a testament to Dr. Akukwe's significant role in organized efforts to convince the United States government and other Western countries to save lives in Africa through targeted HIV/AIDS interventions in the continent. Using his training in medicine and epidemiology, Dr Akukwe pioneered the use of verifiable background data as a powerful instrument of advocacy for AIDS remedial efforts in Africa.

Dr. Akukwe's writings on HIV/AIDS, TB and Malaria continue to have lasting influence on policy makers in the West and Africa. On many occasions, senior policy makers in the United States and Africa informed me how specific articles by Dr. Akukwe moved them to take action on key HIV/AIDS issues. Dr. Akukwe believes the best way to influence policy makers in Africa and the West on HIV/AIDS in Africa is to provide solid background materials on key aspects of the epidemic and to provide a possible road map for remedial efforts. Dr. Akukwe's articulation of Tuberculosis and Malaria as possible "forgotten diseases" despite high morbidity and mortality rates in Africa certainly caught the attention of senior policy makers in the public and private sector.

Thus, the second significant contribution of Dr. Akukwe to AIDS remedial efforts is the need to resolve strategic options for intervention by linking background information/epidemiology of the epidemic with a possible roadmap for specific policy, program or logistics action. From his background as a senior faculty member in various universities in public health, health services management and business, Dr. Akukwe believes that most policy makers will act, within limits set by financial and technical constraints, if they have enough background information on key issues and specific pointers to viable intervention options. Dr. Akukwe's utilization of the population data of jurisdictions in the United States to describe the level of HIV/AIDS impact in Africa caught the attention of policy makers and advocacy organizations.

As you will note in the essays selected for this publication, I co-authored many HIV/AIDS documents on Africa with Dr. Akukwe. These documents combined with the ground-breaking prestige brought to AIDS advocacy for Africa in the United States by the Chairman of the CFA, former Congressman Ron Dellums and the Vice Chairman, former Congressman and former Secretary Jack Kemp paved the way for CFA and other organizations successful advocacy efforts on HIV/AIDS in the United States.

Dr. Chinua's Akukwe's commitment to strong, prosperous Africa is evident in his writings. I can testify that this strong commitment is also evident in his personal interactions. Dr. Akukwe has an abiding faith on Africa's renaissance. However, like all those trained in science, he is a realist that understands that Africans must be on the driver's seat of development issues in the continent. He strongly believes that the HIV/AIDS, TB and Malaria epidemic in Africa is an opportunity for African governments and institutions to reform their politics, economic policies, governance and health systems so that a multi-sectoral response to the epidemic could become possible at local, state, national, sub-regional and continental levels. As noted in many of the essays in this book, HIV/AIDS has left indelible impact on virtually every sector of national economies in Africa and continues to strain the famed extended family system in Africa.

The message of this book is that time is of the essence. Millions of Africans have died of AIDS. Millions more will die this year, next year, and so on. Yet we have lifesaving medicines and preventive know-how to make a difference. We should not allow this situation to continue.

After more than 30 years of working on African issues, in the continent and in the United States, I believe that if enough individuals, governments, the private sector and the civil society raise their commitment for HIV/AIDS, TB and Malaria remedial efforts in Africa, future generations of Africans will be spared untimely death from AIDS. I commend Dr. Akukwe for his past contributions on AIDS remedial efforts in Africa. I hope this book is a reaffirmation of Dr. Akukwe's continued participation in HIV/ AIDS remedial efforts. It is my belief that this book will encourage other individuals and organizations that have made immeasurable contributions to the fight against HIV/AIDS in Africa, to do more. Finally, this book should inspire younger men and women, still mulling their career options, to join the international effort to stop AIDS, TB and Malaria in Africa.

Melvin Foote
President and Chief Executive Officer
Constituency for Africa,
Washington, DC

INTRODUCTION

HIV/AIDS is a worldwide menace, but more than 60 per cent of individuals living with HIV/AIDS are Africans. At least 25.8 million Africans currently live with HIV/AIDS. An estimated 3.2 million Africans contracted HIV in 2005. For more than 2.4 million African adults and children, 2005 was their last year on earth as they died of AIDS. Rightly, the world's concern about the HIV/AIDS pandemic is concentrated on Africa above all. It is a terrible extra affliction for a continent that had more than enough problems without it, especially the widespread poverty and deprivation which, in fact, aggravate the AIDS crisis in Africa.

For several years, as an African living in Washington, I have been adding my voice to the efforts to arouse awareness and concern, especially in the USA, about the urgency of halting the ravages of AIDS in Africa. Now my various articles and speeches on the subject are brought together in this volume, as essays intended to keep this urgent issue before the public.

There is no cure for AIDS as yet. But antiretroviral therapy (ART) can prolong the lives of individuals living with AIDS, and it does so in the USA and other Western countries. In the early 1980s it was HIV/AIDS in America that was constantly in the world's headlines; now, it is HIV/AIDS in Africa. Why?

Not only are the numbers of individuals living with HIV/AIDS far greater in Africa, but, unlike the situation in the West, AIDS is a sentence of death in Africa. Access to lifesaving anti retroviral therapy (ART) changed HIV/AIDS to a mostly clinically manageable and chronic illness in the West, with death rates cut by more than two-thirds since the mid1990s in the United States. In Africa, access to lifesaving medicines is the exception rather than the rule - and yet they all could have access to it.

Other issues loom large. More than 90 percent of Africans living with HIV/AIDS are unaware of their status. They can unwittingly infect other people. Millions of African children 15 years or less have lost their mothers or both parents to AIDS over the last two decades. By 2010, at least 18 million AIDS orphans will be living in

Africa. Today, there is very little organized effort to support these children or meet their health, educational and social welfare needs. Pregnant women in Africa account for more than 90 percent of maternal-to-child transmission of HIV in the world. Yet inexpensive medications exist that can cut maternal-to-child transmissions by more than 50 percent. I can go on and on.

Africa without doubt is the epicenter of HIV/AIDS. Individuals and families infected and affected by HIV/AIDS usually fight the illness with limited local, national or international support. It is a lonely fight and families spend their meager resources to keep a breadwinner alive. Teenagers and young men and women fight their own battles to avoid contracting HIV/AIDS. The epidemic is deep rooted in many countries across Africa, and, current remedial efforts remain tentative, at best. For some families, remedial efforts are too little or too late.

My essays in **Part I of this book, "The Impact of HIV/AIDS in Africa"**, highlight the grim situation in a continent where about a third of the adult populations of several countries - Zimbabwe, Botswana, Lesotho and Swaziland - are infected with HIV, and rates are very high in many other countries, especially in Eastern and Southern Africa but in other regions also. These essays not only discuss the impact of HIV/AIDS but also suggest possible remedial strategies. I also highlight the impact of HIV/AIDS on Africa civil service in another essay. The effects are all the worse in that AIDS strikes down the youngest and fittest most of all. Life expectancy is now 40 years or less in nine African countries hit hard by AIDS, reversing decades of progress. It leaves countless acres of farmland without fit young men and women to do the vital agricultural work that had largely fed the continent through multiple generations despite the effect of famine, wars and diseases; HIV/AIDS is one cause of the agricultural crisis in Zimbabwe. Teachers and other qualified workers are struck down in great numbers; African armies are decimated by the epidemic. Industries in South Africa, the most industrialized country of Africa and the one with the largest number of individuals living with HIV/AIDS, are severely hit by AIDS killing their skilled workers; at least 28 percent of miners in South Africa are believed to live with HIV/AIDS. Basic production in many countries is being set back, or could soon be set back by HIV/AIDS in Africa.

In my essay on the "Feminization of AIDS" I highlight the disproportionate impact of AIDS on women. For every ten men who suffer from it, twelve women harbor the virus. Women suffer particularly because of poverty, deep-rooted cultural norms and widely tolerated male misbehavior. I stress in that essay the need for change in some widespread aspects of African culture. The spread of HIV/AIDS can only be encouraged by the way in which the "big man" assumes he can have any woman who takes his fancy, and the common abuse of positions of authority - as teachers or employers - to demand sexual favors. HIV/AIDS in Africa is a largely a sexually transmitted virus although concern is growing about high rates of infection from individuals injecting themselves with illicit substances from dirty needles.

Part II of this document discusses the response of African governments and institutions to the unfolding tragedy of HIV/AIDS. A major focus of the essays in this section is the fact that no external organization will do for Africa what it must do for itself. African leaders need to take charge of remedial efforts in the continent. African institutions and professional associations need to work together to ensure the establishment of Africa's HIV/AIDS priorities. These priorities should be at the forefront of the relationship between the continent and its bilateral and multilateral organizations and other external partners.

As a major sexually transmitted virus, HIV is forcing reluctant leaders in various fields to tackle the hitherto taboo subject of sex and sexual practices. In Africa, it is unfamiliar territory for political, religious and community leaders as they speak out in public about events that occur in the most private moments. As expected, it has not been easy.

For individuals at risk or already engaging in high risk behavior, the task at hand is not easy, either. These individuals must take on one of the most difficult and terrifying steps in an African society, that is, to discuss with strangers concerns about their most intimate affairs. We expect these already embarrassed individuals to come forward for voluntary testing and counseling, to inform their loved of their HIV status, and, to collaborate with their partners in changing risky behaviors. In the midst of poverty and other socioeconomic struggles in the continent, are we asking too much of Africans who are at risk of contracting HIV? Additionally, HIV preventive programs in Africa face significant challenges as populations at risk evaluate the sincerity of the messengers of preventive messages, evaluate the cultural appropriateness of preventive messages, and analyze the practicalities of personal behavioral changes in their lifestyle and social mores.

Despite the aforementioned challenges, it is a race against time to ensure that Africans and other peoples around the world over-come their discomfort in utilizing services and programs that can help them avoid contracting HIV. It is also a race against time to link those living with the disease with timely clinical care and social support. Every individual who is currently HIV negative has the ultimate responsibility to keep it that way. As I stress throughout these essays, Africans have the primary responsibility for acting against the HIV/AIDS scourge in their continent. African govern-ments have very great responsibilities, for improving their health systems, services and programs. However, Africa cannot do this alone.

In one essay I urge that the development efforts which African leaders hope to pursue under NEPAD (the New Partnership for Africa's Development) must include specific implementation steps against HIV/AIDS. Unless the spread of AIDS is halted all devel-opment efforts will be undermined. Already, according to the World Bank and UNAIDS, HIV/AIDS in the hardest hit countries of Africa is directly responsible for an annual loss of 0.5-1.2 percent of GDP - though Africa must achieve a growth rate of 7 percent to meet the United Nations Millennium Development Goal (MDG) of halving poverty levels by 2015.

Some African countries by the size of their economy and intel-lectual capital should take the lead role in mobilizing support for AIDS remedial efforts throughout the continent. The unfortunate controversies over AIDS policies and programs in South Africa a few years ago robed the continent of a natural leader in AIDS re-medial efforts. The political instability in Nigeria prior to the advent of current civilian government in 1999 shortchanged Africa of that country's natural, leadership role on HIV/AIDS issues. Nigeria's current economic problems and its delicate political system did not give much room for vigorous and sustained leadership on HIV/AIDS in the continent. In a cruel irony, South Africa and Nigeria are not only the two countries with the largest concentration of individuals living with HIV/AIDS in Africa, but with the exception of India, in the world as well.

The decision by South Africa and Nigeria governments to provide ART to their citizens, despite the current modest scale of programs in both countries represent a remarkable chance for strong continental leadership on HIV/AIDS. South Africa, in particular, as I urge in one essay in Part I need to provide comprehensive preventive and treatment programs for its people, and, assist many other African countries, especially its neighbors to fight HIV/AIDS. Many African countries need to step up their efforts, including countries in North Africa where current low levels can easily change without eternal vigilance and strong political support. For Nigeria, it is a race against time because of its huge population and the high rates of poverty; I argue in one essay that the Nigerian government must do more.

Nobody will help Africa unless it is ready to help itself. That must always be borne in mind; as I warn in one essay, it must be remembered all the more as some of the world's attention is turned towards the spread of AIDS in Asia and Eastern Europe. But however vital it is for Africa to help itself, it cannot do so unaided. UNAIDS has estimated that a least 80 percent of the resources required to combat AIDS in Africa must come from external resources.

In Part III, I discuss whether TB and malaria, two conditions with significant morbidity and mortality rates in Africa are forgotten diseases. It is right to devote the new Global Fund to three major killer diseases, for in the proper concern about HIV/AIDS the deadly ravages of malaria and tuberculosis should not be forgotten. One of the essays in Part III serves to remind Westerners - ordinary Africans do not need reminding - that those older diseases are still a major threat. In Africa about 900,000 people die of malaria every year, and up to 40 per cent of an African country's public health expenditure can be devoted to malaria treatment alone. The efforts of the Roll Back Malaria Initiative and the STOP TB Partnership need to be supplemented from an adequate Global Fund. In another accompanying essay in Part III, I outline how TB and malaria programs could be integrated into HIV/AIDS remedial efforts. For those other diseases there are at least proven clinical regimen that could be sustained over a long time. For AIDS there is no known cure. An effective HIV vaccine is at least seven years away. It is important, however, to investigate every claim of "cure" or reduced HIV transmission as the race against time, continues.

Part IV is entitled "AIDS and the Response of International Organizations." HIV/AIDS certainly is a global phenomenon, and in this age of globalization every part of the world, for reasons of sheer self-interest, needs to help cope with AIDS in other parts of the world. The need for such cooperation is supported by Africa and Western governments. However, words must be matched with funds and necessary action on the ground in recipient countries. Not only money is needed, but also effective organization, robust management systems, and, clever logistics strategies; one essay in Part II reproduces proposals I and my colleague made in 2001 for the Global Trust Fund then being considered for international efforts against HIV/AIDS. To provide the necessary finance, the Global Fund for AIDS, Malaria and Tuberculosis was eventually set up. It is remarkable that the early structure of the Global Fund bore close semblance to our proposal. The Global Fund is a very welcome step, but it is essential that its funded programs should be sufficiently large and sustained over a long period of time.

The G8 summit of 2005, at Gleneagles in Scotland, produced a welcome commitment to provide funds for "universal access" to anti-retroviral therapy by 2010 for those in need. But that summit also reaffirmed the aid donors' concerns about "governance" in aid recipient countries. The urgent need for external aid to combat HIV/AIDS should galvanize African governments to answer those concerns. This should not be seen as submission to unreasonable Western demands. It is Africans who suffer from the corruption, discrimination and misgovernment that worry the bilateral and multilateral aid donors. Such things hamper anti-AIDS efforts among other things; civil wars, in particular, wreck those efforts by destroying health services and putting large numbers of people at the mercy of soldiers and irregular combatants. At the same time, it is important to implement comprehensive, verifiable bilateral and multilateral initiatives in areas of need in Africa.

The need for global pharmaceutical companies to respond with agility and in a timely manner to the unique needs of individuals living with HIV/AIDS is more urgent as more than 6 million people now qualify for clinical treatment with ART worldwide. Global pharmaceutical companies have enough ART to meet the needs of those who need them. For Africans living with HIV/AIDS, timely access to ART is a matter of life and death. Africans living with HIV/AIDS must be helped to have ready access to ART.

An important issue here is that of patents and control over production of medicines by research pharmaceutical companies. Unless developing countries can be allowed under World Trade Organization (WTO) rules to produce their own generic drugs, arrange to buy their own generics or set up licensing agreements to meet the needs of those who will die if readily available drugs do not get to them on time, it would be difficult for research pharmaceutical companies to escape close scrutiny and criticism from civil society organizations and other advocates for unimpeded access to lifesaving medicines. Fortunately developing countries obtained the green light for doing this at the WTO's Doha summit in 2001, on which I and my colleagues include a short comment in Part II. This concession was made in a declaration on application of the Agreement on Trade-Related Aspects of Intellectual Property Rights (the TRIPS Agreement).

Africa and its Western partners continue to collaborate on development in initiatives. Western nations have raised their financial and technical contribution to HIV/AIDS remedial efforts in Africa. However, the need remains overwhelming and time is of the essence.

I emphasize the need for more Western support for AIDS remedial efforts in Africa in my essays in **Part V, "The AIDS Crisis in Africa and the Responsibility of the West."** This section begins with an article I wrote in 2001 with a colleague asking how the West will react if the huge numbers of infected and dying people occur in North America or Europe. A lot has happened since we wrote that article. Today, the major challenge is having enough funds to support promising HIV/AIDS remedial efforts in Africa and other developing regions. In the next article in this section, I discuss the current looming funding crisis in HIV/AIDS remedial efforts as a critical issue that deserves the close attention of rich, Western governments. In this essay, I indicated that the Global Fund was (at the time in question) short of $700 million for 2005 and would require an additional $2.9 billion in 2006 and $3.3 billion in 2007.

In the next essay, I discuss my certain belief in the earliest days of the Bush Administration in 2001 that HIV/AIDS will become a major foreign policy priority of the new administration. At that time, in early 2001, it appeared that Africa and HIV/AIDS were not high on the agenda of the new administration. Subsequent events proved that a disease that afflicted the most productive segments of the population sooner rather than later will get the attention of policy makers in the richest nation on earth.

Concentrating particularly on the United States, I noted that as the remaining superpower, it must lead the global effort to fight one of the most devastating health and development challenges in the history of mankind. I am particularly happy that President Bush responded to the growing calls for sustained United States engagement and leadership on Global HIV/AIDS issues by the worldwide initiative to spend $15 billion over five years in 15 countries, 12 in Africa, to deal with HIV/AIDS, TB and malaria. While that marked a huge step forward, more is needed. Not only do the world's richer countries, including the richest of all, need to devote more funds to direct efforts to combat HIV/AIDS; there must also be, at the same time, concrete initiatives to help African countries relieve the prevailing poverty in the continent.

That Africa requires sustained international assistance is not a matter of speculation. In Africa, about 300 million people are estimated to live on $1 a day. At least 75 per cent of people lack basic sanitation and access to clean drinking water in Africa. The economy of Africa is about the size of the national economy of Belgium. The continent is unlikely to trade its way out of poverty in the near future as farmers face comprehensive agricultural trade barriers and subsidies in the United States and Europe.

To overcome poverty Africans must be in the driver's seat regarding design and implementation of programs, but the West can help especially with debt relief. I urge in particular that countries with more than 5 percent HIV prevalence should have one hundred percent debt cancellation, with the savings invested in verifiable programs in health, education and social services. The consequences of HIV/AIDS spreading at current rates will be devastating and will extend beyond individual African states and beyond the shores of Africa.

One devastating effect already widespread is the large number of AIDS orphans, commonly being brought up by overburdened and very poor grandparents after the death of one or more of their parents. Many children are born with HIV in addition, and most will die within the first few years of life. Even those who are born healthy have very bleak and unpromising lives as AIDS orphans as the continent's much vaunted extended family system come under increasing strain from sickness and untimely deaths of men and women in their most productive years. The UNAIDS estimates that by 2010, at least 18 million AIDS orphans will live in Africa if the present state of infection and death continues unabated. As these deprived and embittered children grow up many will be willing recruits for irregular forces in any new civil war that comes along. The pandemic is a threat to peace in Africa, and the rest of the world cannot ignore such threats.

It is not only governments in the West that I urge to help avert such threats. In some of the essays in Part IV I urge African Americans to help as individuals, perhaps by spending a year helping anti-AIDS efforts in Africa. I make that appeal not only to the long established American community of African descent, but also to what is called the "New Diaspora" - the millions of Africans who have settled in the USA and Western Europe in recent decades. These include large numbers of highly qualified people who could devote some time in helping anti-AIDS programs back in Africa, even if they do not start a reversal of the regrettable "brain drain" by going home permanently to serve the home continent. This appeal is not only made to health workers, though they are urgently needed, especially as in Africa, as many have left the continent and many others have suffered disproportionately from AIDS. A survey in South Africa found 16 per cent of health workers to be living with HIV/AIDS. HIV/AIDS remedial effort in Africa requires the active participation of multi-sectoral teams working on identified problems and challenges.

As I look toward the future on AIDS remedial efforts, I call in Part VI for a complete rethink of global HIV/AIDS strategies. A rethink of global HIV/AIDS should include consolidation of service delivery in recipient countries; mobilizing available technical, financial and logistical resources to provide timely preventive, clinical and support care; and, ending ideological squabbles that delay implementation of lifesaving programs. **A rethink of AIDS remedial effort is critical as the** rate of HIV transmission shows no sign of slowing down and death from AIDS is not decreasing. Individuals and families battling HIV/AIDS, despite the valiant efforts of domestic and international agencies and organization, have very little contact with any component of ongoing domestic or international remedial efforts. As resources are scarce and the needs are multiplying, the consolidation of international HIV/AIDS programs in recipient country levels is of outmost importance Recipient countries are increasingly bearing the burden of too many external partners performing exactly the same functions or providing similar services. In addition, I proposed to the American Bar Association (ABA) that its members could help with legal problems connected with the pandemic - in the area of women's rights, for example, ending gender inequity issues, discrimination and stigma.

I propose with some of my colleagues a new international volunteer corps for help with HIV/AIDS prevention and treatment programs in Africa. A rethink of HIV/AIDS global strategies will require stepping out of the box and embracing new challenges; motivating professional organizations that have not had pivotal roles so far in AIDS remedial effort to provide technical and financial support; mobilizing new resources in public and private sectors; and, galvanizing individuals and organizations to go beyond the call of duty to devote their time and resources to making a difference, one person at a time in AIDS hardest-hit countries.

These essays do not cover all aspects of this important topic. But I hope that they will contribute to increased awareness in Africa, Europe and the United States of this great menace to the world that at this point in time is laying a siege in Africa.

PART I

The Impact of HIV/AIDS in Africa

1

THE IMPACT OF HIV/AIDS IN AFRICA

(November 2005)

I begin this section with a short commentary on the impact of HIV/AIDS in Africa as known in November 2005. Subsequent articles highlight known impact of HIV/AIDS in the continent as at the time I wrote cited articles.

In 2005, the UNAIDS estimated that 25.8 million people live with HIV/AIDS in Africa, accounting for 64 percent of all individuals worldwide living with the condition. UNAIDS estimates that 3.2 million Africans became infected with HIV in 2005, and, 2.4 million men, women and children lost their battle to AIDS. Two African nations, South Africa and Nigeria have two of the three countries in the world with the largest concentration of individuals living with HIV/AIDS (India is the non-African country). More than 5 and 3 million people respectively live with HIV/AIDS in South Africa and Nigeria. Southern Africa continues to bear the brunt of the pandemic, accounting for more than 30 percent of all individuals living with HIV/AIDS worldwide despite representing only 2 percent of the global population.

The adult prevalence rate of HIV/AIDS in Africa is 7.2 percent, compared to prevalence rates of 0.7 percent in North America, 0.3 percent in Western and Central Europe, 1.6 percent in the Caribbean and 0.6 percent in Latin America. More than 90 percent of all Africans living with HIV/AIDS are unaware of their HIV status. Levels of knowledge about HIV transmission and risk factors remain low in many African countries. In some conflict-prone areas such as Southern Sudan, level of knowledge is even much lower as communities emerge from isolated conflict zones and refugee camps.

African women remain at major risk of contracting HIV. More than three-fourth (77 percent) of all women living with HIV/AIDS worldwide are African women. In 2005, thirteen and half million Africa women were living with HIV/AIDS. This is about 57 percent of all HIV/AIDS cases in Africa, the highest rate of infection among women in all regions of the world. Pregnant women in Africa account for more than 90 percent of all mother-to-child transmission of HIV in the world. In Swaziland, according to UNAIDS, pregnant women had HIV prevalence rates of 43 percent in 2004. Astonishingly, young women in many parts of Africa have limited knowledge of the risk factors of HIV transmission. The UNAIDS reports that a recent survey of 24 countries in Sub-Saharan Africa revealed that at least two-thirds of girls and young women ages 15-24 did not show comprehensive knowledge of the risk factors for HIV transmission. Two out of every five pregnant women were living with HIV/AIDS in six countries in southern Africa: Botswana, Lesotho, Namibia, South Africa, Swaziland and Zimbabwe.

Although more than 80 percent of individuals living with HIV/AIDS in developing countries such as Argentina, Brazil, Chile and Cuba are on ART, only one in ten Africans, at any point in time, are on ART despite urgent clinical need. Less than 5 percent of AIDS orphans are on any form of social support in Africa. AIDS has the capacity to reduce national GDP by 0.5-1.0 percent in hardest-hit countries. No sector, public or private, is spared with HIV/AIDS. Life expectancy in nine Africa countries is now less than 40 years, figures last seen four decades ago in these countries. HIV/AIDS is now accepted as a major development crisis in Africa.

2

THE IMPACT OF HIV/AIDS ON THE CIVIL SERVICE IN AFRICA*

(November 2005)

I thank the National Academy of Public Administration and the Africa Working Group for this opportunity to share my insights on the impact of HIV/AIDS on Africa's civil service. The Africa Working Group of the Academy under the leadership of Professor Sy Murray deserves credit for its focus on HIV/AIDS in Africa.

The civil service in Africa is unique for many reasons. First, an indigenous civil service is fairly young in Africa since most countries in the continent became politically independent in the last four decades.

Second, the civil service in many African countries represents the best and the brightest of their generation since government is still the predominant employer of labor.

Third, a typical civil servant in Africa, no matter his or her grade or monthly pay is responsible for the upkeep of more than 10 individuals. This responsibility ranges from the needs of immediate family members to the support of the extended family.

Fourth, civil servants are leaders in their communities and hometowns, with influence exceeding what many in industrialized societies may comprehend. These civil servants are the natural opinion leaders of their communities, and, are often relied upon to attract government programs and services to their communities.

Fifth, top civil servants in many poor African countries represent years of significant investments in education and in-service training that may not be immediately replaceable.

Finally, in communities and environments where poverty is the rule rather the exception, civil servants such as teachers, nurses and agricultural extension workers are crucial to an impoverished community's hopes to train their young, keep them alive and feed them properly to become effective leaders of tomorrow.

Consequently, extended illness or death of a civil servant in Africa has major repercussions. The immediate family will likely spend its meager resources trying to keep the breadwinner alive. Extended family members may no longer go to school as funds for school fees go toward keeping the breadwinner alive. The community may lose a valuable contact in government and policymaking circles. A national government may be left reeling from loss of highly experienced but difficult to replace worker.

Today in many African countries, HIV/AIDS is having extraordinary impact on the workforce. According to the United Nations International Labor Organization (ILO), a minimum of 26 million people worldwide living with HIV/AIDS are in the workforce, with at least two-thirds of them living in Africa. By the end of 2005, ILO estimates that worldwide more than two million workers, two-thirds of them living in Africa, will be too sick to go to work because of AIDS. In Uganda, ILO estimates that more than 50 percent of all teachers are living with HIV/AIDS. Tanzania loses 100 primary school teachers every month to AIDS. At least one million children in Africa have lost their teachers to AIDS. In Malawi, AIDS deaths among the civil service increased tenfold between 1990 and 2000. In many parts of Africa, the biggest threat is no longer neighboring armies but HIV/AIDS in its rank and file. The police force and other paramilitary organizations in Africa are dealing with high rates of HIV/AIDS with devastating impact on performance and morale. By 2020, HIV/AIDS will cause between 10 and 30 percent reduction in the labor force of AIDS hard hit countries in Africa. For Nigeria and South Africa, with large concentration of individuals living with the HIV/AIDS, the effect is likely to be higher.

It is also important to note that the impact of HIV/AIDS is not restricted to government bureaucracies. In the private sector in Africa, the effect is equally devastating. According to the ILO, a survey of 26 firms in South Africa showed a 13.0 percent HIV prevalence in the manufacturing sector. In the same survey, 20.4 percent of all contract workers were living with HIV/AIDS, 14.8

percent of unskilled workers were infected with HIV and 4.1 percent of managerial cadres were living with HIV. The rates are higher in Botswana and Zambia. In many instances, businesses reportedly hire two or more individuals for the same position as a hedge against the inevitable absence from work or death from AIDS.

HIV/AIDS is a disease of the workforce in Africa. Unfortunately, workplace initiatives that address HIV/AIDS are yet to become a mainstream public sector issue in the continent. A workplace HIV/AIDS initiative on HIV/AIDS should include preventive programs, testing and counseling services, clinical care, support care, and timely transition benefits care for the families of workers who die of AIDS. The workplace initiative should also improve legal protections for workers living with HIV/AIDS. In addition, in Africa, a workplace HIV/AIDS initiative should include programs for extended family members and outreach services to the communities where workers live.

In my work with the UN International Labor Organization Program on HIV/AIDS, it became clear that workplace initiatives on HIV/AIDS should become a top priority of African governments to ensure timely access to preventive, clinical and support care for workers. It also became apparent that African countries needed to enact or enforce laws against employment discrimination due to HIV status. Laws protecting confidentiality of medical records need to be strengthened as an incentive for workers at risk of contracting HIV to come forward for testing and counseling.

HIV/AIDS in the work place also calls for an end to the usual adversarial relationship between management and labor unions. Since HIV/AIDS is now an emergency problem in the workforce, senior civil servants in Africa, political leaders and labor union leaders need to work together to minimize the impact of HIV/AIDS in the workforce. The key is to prevent new HIV infection, keep infected workers as productive as possible and provide timely support care for their families if the workers are too sick to work or die of AIDS.

I thank you for the opportunity to address this plenary session.

* Invited Presentation by Dr. Chinua Akukwe at the 2005 National Academy of Public Administration Conference, Pentagon City, Virginia, United States, November 28, 2005

3

FEMINIZATION OF AIDS: TEN UNAVOIDABLE CHOICES FOR AFRICAN LEADERS*

(March 9, 2005)

The UNAIDS report on the HIV/AIDS pandemic highlights the growing rates of infection among women worldwide. Women now account for nearly 50 percent of all individuals living with HIV/AIDS worldwide. However, in Africa, the situation is more ominous. Almost 57 percent of all individuals living with HIV/AIDS in Africa are women. For Africans aged 15-24 living with HIV/AIDS, women account for 76 percent of all infections. In South Africa, Zambia and Zimbabwe, young women aged 15-24 have rates of infection that are between three and six times that of their male peers.

The so called feminization of AIDS appears to be in full swing in Africa. The key question is whether African leaders and elite are ready to make hard choices that would slow down the rate of infection among women. I briefly review these choices. The key is to focus on practical solutions to a problem that can only get worse if nothing is done.

First, are African leaders and governments ready to mount a comprehensive and sustained information, education and communication campaign against risk-behaving practices of men that put women at risk of HIV infection? I am not aware of any African country that is currently implementing a sustained, nationwide campaign against sugar daddies, the use of large sums of money by male clients to encourage sex workers to engage in unprotected sex, the rape of young girls by school teachers, the molestation of young girls by family members and the molestation of street children. African men who have disposable income are at the root of sexual networking in various communities that spread HIV, according to UNAIDS.

Second, are African leaders and governments ready to address cultural practices that may put women at a disadvantage in the fight against HIV/AIDS? These practices include lack of proactive opportunities for women to discuss sexual mores and risks with their husbands, cultural expectations of subservience in sexual matters, the culture of wife inheritance after widowhood, and the lack of property rights for widows or single women even when they have to take care of small children.

Third, are African leaders and governments ready to invest for the long term in female education? According to the latest data from the World Bank, 45 percent of women aged 15 and above in Sub-Sahara Africa are illiterate. While 94 percent of boys are enrolled in primary school only 81 percent of girls are in school. For starters, primary and secondary school education should be free in Africa to allow young people, including girls, to have a head start in life. It is also important for African women to have increased access to university education, especially those from poor families. However, to ensure quality education for African women, African governments and rich nations such as the United States and other Western democracies should provide increased, targeted development assistance for Africa. Rich nations and multilateral institutions such as the World Bank and the International Monetary Fund should provide comprehensive debt relief for Africa with a major condition that significant portions of the savings from debt relief should go toward social welfare programs such as financing of education initiatives for girls and young women.

Fourth, are African leaders and governments ready to create enabling environments for empowering African women? Limited economic choices and opportunities constrict the capacity of African women to negotiate safer personal behavior, including sexual relations. Although African women are major sources of economic wealth in many rural parts of Africa, these women have limited control over their generated income owing to cultural taboos and traditional practices. African governments should end cultural practices that deny women the right to benefit from their toil and labor. It is also important for African governments to create micro-credit facilities for enterprising rural women so that they can become stable, small-scale entrepreneurs and accumulate disposable income. Women with disposable income are likely to make better personal choices for themselves and their children.

Fifth, can African leaders and governments create political space for women? Regardless of many official statistics that cite token numbers of national ministers and top government officials that are women, I believe that in order to fight AIDS, women must be in decision making organs in local and state governments throughout Africa, and also have leadership roles in key national government institutions such as the ministries of finance, national planning and justice. In addition, African women should be in decision making positions in civil society, local chambers of commerce and local youth organizations that directly interface with the grassroots. It is important to state without equivocation that female representation in national cabinets in Africa should go beyond the obligatory "Ministry of Women or Gender Affairs."

Sixth, are African leaders and governments ready to create necessary legal climate and framework that protect women from discrimination and lack of due process? UNAIDS estimates that more than 50 percent of African countries do not have legal statutes that outlaw discrimination against individuals living with HIV/AIDS. In Africa, according to UNAIDS, fear of an HIV test among women, including pregnant mothers, is the beginning of wisdom, since negative societal consequences and uncertain future may lie ahead if they test positive. For women living with HIV/AIDS, the prospect of dealing with family, community and government indifference and sometimes hostility can be insurmountable. Legal reforms on rape, sexual molestations, domestic violence, favors-for-forced sexual relations, property rights, and ownership of business are crucial in the fight against feminization of HIV/AIDS.

Seventh, are African leaders and governments ready to invest in public health services that are friendly and accessible to women? National spending on public health services is low in Africa, about US$30 per capita, according to the World Bank. Women face formidable challenges in accessing public health services for conditions such as sexually transmitted diseases and tuberculosis that are important facilitators of HIV transmission. Privacy and confidentiality are rare in African health institutions, according to UNAIDS. Societal stigma is common when women become linked to sexually transmitted diseases. In addition, fear of violence may keep women from utilizing HIV preventive services or even showing up for AIDS clinical care, according to UNAIDS. It is important for the international community to support African nations that seek to implement female friendly health systems and programs.

Eighth, are African leaders ready to position gender issues as a major priority of international development assistance? Declarations, statements and formal speeches about gender issues should be coupled with specific policy and program initiatives to end gender inequities in Africa. African leaders, continent-wide institutions and civil society should make gender equity a cardinal feature of their relationship with bilateral and multilateral agencies. There is a tendency to point to token appointments of women to prominent positions as celebratory signs of progress on gender issues in Africa. While this is important, the focus should be on hundreds of millions of African women who toil away anonymously, unsung and uncelebrated despite their significant contributions to the economy of the continent. In particular, African governments should make ending gender inequity a top priority of their partnership with donor agencies. A good measure of serious commitment is the proportion of resources requested by African governments to deal with gender inequities in proposals sent to donor agencies. National budgets should also reflect increased resources devoted to ending gender inequities and creating income-generating opportunities for women.

Ninth, can African leaders lead the fight against sexual violence against women? Official, societal and personal silence on sexual violence against women is deafening in many parts of Africa. In particular, perpetrators target female teenagers in some parts of Africa, thereby potentially setting off a chain of events that may leave the young women not only emotionally scarred for life but also in the ever possible risk and danger of HIV/AIDS. To end sexual violence, African governments would have to deny perpetrators of sexual violence political, economic, legal and social sanctuary. Zero legal tolerance against sexual violence should be enforced and perpetrators subjected to the long arm of the law. Women should be encouraged to come forward with cases of sexual violence and the society should treat them with compassion while the legal system runs its course.

Tenth, African leaders and governments must win the battle against widespread poverty in the continent. Poverty is a major reason why individuals, including women, knowingly engage in high risk behavior that facilitates the spread of HIV. Feminization of HIV/AIDS is closely intertwined with poverty and harsh living conditions. African leaders and governments should create opportunities for poor women to escape poverty through sustainable macroeconomic policies that improve their vocational skills, provide access to literacy programs, provide incentives for self employment and allow them to accumulate capital and properties. Rich nations, including the United States, should work closely with Africa leaders in this regard. Comprehensive debt relief, increased access to trade for African farmers and businesses, and comprehensive micro-credit programs are also critical policy issues that rich nations can assist African nations as part of a comprehensive fight against poverty.

Conclusion

Efforts to end the feminization of AIDS in Africa must be African-based and African-implemented. For the African woman at the receiving end of HIV/AIDS, the solution lies principally in changing societal beliefs and practices within her family, community, country and the continent. The solution to gender inequities lies in the capacity of African governments to confront societal beliefs and practices that wittingly or unwittingly put women at risk of physical, emotional and mental harm.

The HIV/AIDS epidemic in Africa is exposing deadly consequences of gender inequities. As the toll of HIV/AIDS mounts in Africa and the epidemic gradually assumes a feminine connotation, every policy maker in Africa should work toward the end of all practices that prevent African women from becoming full partners in the titanic struggle ahead. Any serious advocate for comprehensive

AIDS remedial efforts in Africa cannot afford to watch from the sidelines the increasing feminization of AIDS in the continent.

Bibliography

1. UNAIDS (2004). *AIDS Epidemic Update: 2004.* November. Geneva, Switzerland: Author. Available at the UNAIDS website, www.unaids.org This is the latest update on the global AIDS situation and is dedicated to the feminization of AIDS. Data used in this article are available in the PDF format of the update under the following sections and pages: Introduction, pages 2-6; Women and AIDS, pages 7, 9-17 dealing on issues such as gender inequities, problems with accessing preventive and clinical care, power imbalances, fear of violence, lack of property rights, cultural taboo about discussing sexual mores and risks with husbands; Sub-Saharan Africa, pages 19, 23, 24, 27, 28, 29 on issues that affect women in Africa and the impact on the spread of HIV.

2. UNAIDS (2004). *2004 Report on the Global AIDS Epidemic.* July. Geneva, Switzerland: Author. Available at the UNAIDS website, www.unaids.org This document released during the Bangkok AIDS conference in July 2004 contains a collection of information on the epidemic. The PDF format includes an executive summary that also discusses continued discrimination against women and the lack of enabling legislation that outlaws stigma and discrimination against individuals living with HIV/AIDS.

3. World Bank (2004). *African Development Indicators 2004.* Washington, DC: Author. This is widely considered the authoritative database on Africa's development. Data cited in this article are found in pages 320, 322, 323 on healthcare expenditure per capita, illiteracy levels and primary school enrolment. The female economic situation in Africa is shown in page 330 of the document.

4. Chinua Akukwe and Melvin Foote (2001). "HIV/AIDS in Africa: It is Time to End the Killing Fields." *Foreign Policy in Focus,* April.

4

AFRICA: THE IMPLICATIONS OF A GROWING AIDS EPIDEMIC IN ASIA AND EASTERN EUROPE

(August, 2004)

Africa continues to be the epicenter of the HIV/AIDS pandemic with more than 25 million Africans living with the condition. Africa accounts for two-thirds of all HIV/AIDS cases in the world, nearly 80 percent of all deaths, at least 90 percent of maternal-child birth transmissions, and 90 percent of all children who have lost one or both parents to AIDS. However, in the last few years, HIV/AIDS has become a growing concern in Asia and Central Europe. A runaway epidemic in Asia and Central Europe will have major implications for Africa. I discuss these implications.

According to the United Nations organization coordinating the global response to the pandemic (UNAIDS), about 7.4 million Asians are currently living with HIV/AIDS. For the first time, more than one million new infections occurred in Asia in 2003. As this is a region that accounts for 60 percent of humanity, an explosion in new infections will affect a large number of people. Four populous nations in Asia account for the increasing rates of HIV transmission: China, India, Indonesia and Vietnam. In India, at least 5 million individuals live with HIV/AIDS. Growing rates of HIV transmission will be a major headache for industrialized nations that have targeted them for major economic investments. An upsurge in HIV transmission is ongoing in the Russian Federation and the former Soviet-bloc countries of Ukraine, Estonia and Latvia. The number of people living with HIV in Eastern Europe rose from 160,000 in 1995 to 1.3 million today. Most of the infected are less than 30 years of age.

Today, bilateral and multilateral agencies routinely refer to Asia and Eastern Europe as regions with the "fastest" rates of HIV transmission. These agencies citing the huge population at risk are now openly discussing the "global implications" of an "unchecked" epidemic in these regions. For anybody familiar with international development and policy making, these descriptions suggest an impending shift in priorities and strategies.

Specifically for Africa, what are the implications of a shift in HIV/AIDS remedial strategy towards Asia and Eastern Europe?

The first implication is a potential diversion of fiscal resources. Africa, according to UNAIDS, relies on external donors to cover up to 80 percent of the financial outlay for HIV/AIDS remedial efforts. If resources increasingly move to Asia and Eastern Europe, then Africa's response to the epidemic will suffer accordingly. Furthermore, UNAIDS's projection that Africa will account for 43 percent of a global HIV/AIDS expenditure of US$20 billion by 2007 may not necessarily materialize if global attention shifts to Asia and Eastern Europe. Virtually every Africa country including influential South Africa and Nigeria requires sustained external support to meet the needs of individuals infected and affected by HIV/AIDS.

The second implication is that ongoing and largely successful efforts to implement access to life saving HIV/AIDS medicines in Africa may falter as scarce resources move to Asia and Eastern Europe. In addition, recent estimates by UNAIDS that 77 percent of HIV/AIDS expenditure in Asia by 2007 (compared to 35 percent in Africa) will go toward preventive programs may prove attractive to external donors looking for ways to stretch their resources.

The third implication is that many African nations that are just turning the corner on HIV/AIDS remedial efforts may be stranded. The much-heralded success stories in Uganda and Senegal depend on continuous policy and program vigilance that requires fiscal and technical resources. Countries that are turning the corner on HIV/AIDS, such as Zambia and Tanzania, require strong support to maintain the momentum.

The fourth and perhaps gravest implication is a slowdown of preventive programs in Africa. Lack of fiscal and technical resources to implement information, education and communication campaigns against HIV will have major repercussions. A slowdown in support for preventive programs may further drive away high risk behaving individuals. It may also force economic-driven at risk populations, such as commercial sex workers and their patrons, to go underground. Pregnant women may also never know their HIV status and can transmit HIV to their newborn.

Fifth, the army of advocacy organizations and civil society active in the West on accelerated AIDS remedial efforts in Africa may be hard pressed to make a case if China with more than 1 billion people, or India not far behind, continues to record high rates of new infections. The sheer numbers of infected individuals will likely hold the attention of policy makers in the West.

What should African leaders do now to plan for a potential shift of international policy attention to Asia and Eastern Europe as the HIV/AIDS pandemic unfolds? In this regard, time is of the essence. I suggest critical strategic steps.

The key first step is to determine Africa's HIV/AIDS priorities, goals and objectives. I have written in the past on this issue. Africa's HIV/AIDS remedial effort is largely driven by the policy prescriptions of bilateral and multilateral agencies. To overcome this strategic handicap, the African Union (AU), the African Development Bank (ADB) and the United Nations Economic Commission in Africa (ECA) should jointly develop an African response to HIV/AIDS. Under this arrangement, the AU will provide the political and enabling environment for a strong African response. The ADB will provide expertise on project management and also lend its considerable financial muscle. The ECA will come to the table with its widely recognized expertise on policy and operations research. A major outcome of this unprecedented collaboration should be a streamlining of external support for measures against HIV/AIDS in Africa to avoid duplication of functions and services.

Another step is to develop a continental blueprint on how to link accelerated debt relief to verifiable investments on HIV/AIDS and other socio-economic development programs. The current World Bank/IMF Heavily Indebted Poor Countries (HIPC) Initiative on debt relief is yet to have significant impact on Africa's debt burden. According to the latest data from the World Bank, Africa owes US$295 billion to Western creditors. Africa's total external debt per capita is US$358 in a continent where many nations are hard pressed to spend US$4 per capita on healthcare. In developing this blueprint, the experiences of various African countries participating in HIPC should be utilized in developing an Africa Debt Relief-HIV/AIDS Swap initiative. This initiative, in return for accelerated debt relief or outright forgiveness, will commit African nations to verifiable investments on HIV/AIDS remedial efforts, infrastructure development (health, education and other social programs) and good governance.

Another step is to strengthen the capacity of national governments to respond to HIV/AIDS. The key is to develop regional pools of technical experts and make them available to national governments where expertise is lacking. For example, the Economic Community of West African states (ECOWAS) should have a pool of technical experts that should assist member states, as and when due. External donors may also support development of regional expertise on HIV/AIDS.

A critical step is also to mobilize the private sector to provide HIV/AIDS preventive and clinical management services to their workers and immediate families. I once visited a major manu-facturing facility in South Africa and came away hugely impressed by this organization's comprehensive HIV/AIDS program and its outreach services to the local community. The managers of this facility made it clear that it made economic sense to implement a comprehensive remedial effort against HIV/AIDS. The private sector is an untapped resource in HIV/AIDS remedial efforts in Africa.

Finally, the need to revamp or develop community-based health systems in Africa. Today, most internationally directed HIV/AIDS remedial efforts in Africa have very little effect on individuals and families infected or affected by HIV/AIDS. Africa needs to have functional, sustainable community-based health systems that reflect local realities, mobilize target populations, and encourage at-risk groups to come forward for assessment and care. Civil society organizations, especially religious and community entities are critical partners in this regard. The foundation of HIV/AIDS remedial efforts in Africa should be at the community level where most Africans live and die.

In conclusion, it is only a matter of time before the attention of the international community turns towards Asia and Eastern Europe regarding HIV/AIDS. Africa needs to be prepared for this shift. African leaders should take immediate strategic steps to improve the capacity of the continent to respond to the long-term effects of this deadly epidemic. Africa should provide leadership on HIV/AIDS in the continent, even if the epicenter of the pandemic moves to Asia and Eastern Europe.

Selected Bibliography

1. UNAIDS (2004). *2004 Report on the Global AIDS Epidemic*. July. Geneva: Author. This is the source of the data on HIV/AIDS in this article

2. World Bank (2004). *Africa Development Indicators*. Washington, DC: Author. This is the source of the data on economic indicators and the HIPC Initiative in Africa.

5

HIV/AIDS IN AFRICA: CHILDREN INFECTED AND AFFECTED BY THE PANDEMIC*

(April, 2003)

Introduction

Africa is at the crossroads of multiple issues such as poor governance, underdevelopment, conflicts, environmental disasters, economic exploitation, and grinding poverty. However, the HIV/AIDS epidemic is by far the biggest challenge of modern day Africa. With more than 30 million individuals, mostly men and women in the prime of their lives, living with HIV/AIDS in Africa, and less than 5 percent of these individuals having access to lifesaving medicines, the future is not very promising.

African children infected and affected by HIV/AIDS are the ultimate development nightmare for a continent grappling with major socioeconomic problems. According to UNAIDS, every day two thousand infants contract HIV through their mothers throughout the world. At least 95 percent of these infants are born in Africa. Every day, in the entire world, six thousand children lose one or both parents to AIDS. More than 90 percent of these children are Africans. Every day, sixteen hundred children die of AIDS worldwide. At least 90 percent of these dead children are Africans. Today, every child in Southern Africa is 50 percent likely to die of AIDS in his/her lifetime. Today in Africa, 95 percent of pregnant mothers do not have access to health programs that can significantly reduce the incidence of mother-to-child transmission of HIV.

The worst is yet to come. According to UNAIDS, UNICEF and USAID, by 2010, at least 20 million AIDS orphans will live in Africa. This is in a continent where children face the deadly combination of high rates of infant deaths, vaccine preventable deaths, under-five mortality, diarrhoea-related deaths, and death from malaria. It is also a continent where children face major challenges of going to school, staying in school, eating nutritious meals, and having access to adequate sanitation.

African children infected and affected by HIV/AIDS face current and future dangers. These children, as extended family systems become stretched, face the daunting prospects of life on the streets. They also face the ever present dangers of conscription into the sex trade industry and forcible enrolment into private militias and criminal gangs. The education and health needs of these children are unlikely to be met, as shown by the current predicament of Southern Africa's street children. In simple terms, the scenario of 20 million uneducated, street hardened, weather-beaten, and ulti-mately bitter African children will present formidable challenges to constituted governments in the continent by 2010.

Current Remedial Efforts

What are the current policies and programs for children infected and affected by the HIV/AIDS crisis in Africa? Today in Africa, I am not aware of any serious continent-wide, compre-hensive, multi-sectoral policy or program directed at the more than 12 million AIDS orphans in Africa. I am also not aware of any comprehensive, multi-sectoral program directed at children infected and affected by HIV/AIDS in any African country. I am also unaware of any serious, integrated and comprehensive corporate or civil society effort to address the issue of children infected and affected by HIV/AIDS in Africa.

Obviously something is going on in Africa about children infected and affected by HIV/AIDS. I am aware of heroic efforts by small-scale community-based organizations to provide basic support for AIDS orphans in various countries in Africa. I am also aware of the role of faith-based organizations, international agencies, and foundations in addressing pockets of the AIDS orphan problem in Africa. The Gates Foundation initiative on AIDS orphans in selected African countries readily comes to mind. The role of communities and families, most often poor, is also critical in current palliative efforts to address the problems of children infected and affected by HIV/AIDS. Grandparents, especially grandmothers are now major breadwinners for AIDS orphans in many parts of Africa.

It is instructive that as the AIDS orphan crisis grows in Africa, and more children become infected and affected by the epidemic, very little action is underway to meet the needs of these children. Most initiatives in Africa are limited in scope and coverage, and, rarely focused on an index AIDS orphan or a child either infected or affected by the epidemic.

Way Forward

What can be done to remedy the situation? I suggest three basic principles for dealing with children infected and affected by HIV/AIDS in Africa. They are: say no to token or palliative programs - initiatives in Africa should be comprehensive and multi-sectoral in dealing with the needs of infected and affected children; recognize the unique needs of children LIVING with HIV/AIDS and those children AFFECTED by HIV/AIDS; and aggressively prevent transmission of HIV and/or provide antiretroviral therapy to those in need.

To move forward, we must step away from the present comfort zone of providing token, palliative remedies for African children infected and affected by HIV/AIDS. To provide comprehensive multi-sectoral programs, the African Union, the Economic Commission for Africa and the African Development Bank in conjunction with other international partners should develop a continent-wide blueprint for dealing with children infected and affected by HIV/AIDS. This blueprint, while recognizing distinct local and national issues, will set guidelines and parameters for scaled up continent and international remedial efforts. This blueprint should also set guidelines for regional initiatives, for sharing expertise across national boundaries, and for creating opportunities for communities to share lessons learned.

To recognize the unique needs of children infected and/or affected by HIV/AIDS, local, national, continent and international remedial efforts should focus on outcome indicators for an index child. Did this infected child receive his/her lifesaving medicines? Did this affected child complete age-appropriate grade school? Did this infected child meet his/her nutritional needs (for example, through age-appropriate weight gain)? Did this affected child leave the streets and move into decent housing? To meet the challenges of these children, each unique need must be met or considered.

To stop HIV transmission, aggressive information, education and communication campaigns must continue in Africa. Pregnant women in Africa should have access to antiretroviral therapy that can cut maternal transmission in half. Children and adults living with HIV/AIDS should have access to antiretroviral drugs.

Seven years from now, in 2010, Africa will face the prospects of 20 million AIDS orphans and millions of other children infected with HIV. Before 2010, every year, successive cohorts of AIDS orphans will become young adults, the economic and social fulcrum of their societies. No matter our actions or inaction, these children will assume their natural role as the engine room of their societies. Whether these children are socialized, educated, clothed or fed, they will assume their role in the society. The question is what kind of role we expect these children to play in the future. The choice is entirely ours.

---

* Remarks made at the US Congressional Human Rights Caucus (CHRC) Seminar on the Global Challenges of HIV/AIDS: Drawing the Line in Africa, April 2, 2003, Capitol Hill, Washington, DC.

Selected Bibliography

Chinua Akukwe (2002). "HIV/AIDS in Africa: An Integrated Regional Approach." *Africa Notes,* July/August, pages 7-11. Cornell University, Ithaca, New York State.

Peter Piot (2002). *Speech to the United Nations General Assembly Special Session on Children*, United Nations, New York. Geneva: UNAIDS.

UNAIDS (2002). *Report on the Global HIV/AIDS Epidemic*. Geneva: Author.

USAID, UNICEF, UNAIDS (2002). *Children on the Brink 2002*. Washington, DC: USAID.

UNDP (2002). *Millennium Development Goals and the UNDP Role*. New York: Author.

6

HIV/AIDS IN AFRICA: UNRESOLVED
ISSUES AND HARD CHOICES*

(April, 2004)

I thank Congressmen Lantos, Wolff, McDermott, Lee and Leach for their outstanding leadership on human rights issues in the Congress and HIV/AIDS globally, especially in regards to the unfolding AIDS catastrophe in Africa. The Congressional Human Rights Caucus (CHRC) is widely recognized as the conscience of the US Congress on major social issues. As a former member of the International Human Rights Committee of the American Public Health Association, I am aware of the tremendous contributions of Congressman Tom Lantos and Frank Wolff on human rights issues around the world.

HIV/AIDS in Africa remains a major community, national, regional and international challenge. As of today, MOST individuals infected or affected by HIV/AIDS in Africa are on their own, and often go back to their communities to die with little or no clinical/government support.

Virtually all national governments in Africa with high rates of HIV are struggling to find material and human resources to fight the epidemic. Africa, today, is yet to craft a comprehensive regional strategy and program to stop AIDS. On the international scene, despite a flurry of activities by various Western nations and multilateral institutions, very few resources from the West have reached individuals either infected or affected by HIV/AIDS in Africa.

For that young woman with four children dying of AIDS somewhere in Southern Africa, the possibility of Western assistance reaching her or her soon-to-be AIDS orphans is very remote. Yet every Western government, including the United States, is "investing significant" resources in the fight against HIV/AIDS. Every multilateral agency has a "significantly resourced" HIV/AIDS program. Every African leader is "speaking out" against HIV/AIDS, has completed national "action plans" and has "directed" senior cabinet officials to take "charge" of the war on AIDS.

In the 2003 seminar organized by CHRC, I indicated that more than 12 million AIDS orphans in Africa were largely on their own, at the mercy of inclement weather, dangerous African streets, and criminal elements. Since that presentation one year ago, these orphans are yet to receive coordinated regional, sub-regional or national assistance.

The war on AIDS in Africa continues to suffer from a number of unresolved issues.

Access to lifesaving, available medicines is still a mirage and has become a subject of international tug-of-war between powerful rich nations and desperate poor nations. While this needless battle rages, millions of infected and affected Africans continue to die of AIDS. All eyes are now on Randall Tobias and his team in the US $15 billion, five-year AIDS initiative to break this logjam of research versus generic drugs, and make these available and affordable drugs easily accessible to millions of Africans dying of AIDS. The announcement today of South Africa's roll out of its national treatment program is commendable for a nation with the highest number of individuals living with HIV/AIDS, up to 5 million and counting. However, this good news must be juxtaposed with the reality that only about 50,000 people will be on this national program by the end of the year.

Information, education and communication campaigns against HIV transmission in Africa remain unfocused, fragmented, poorly funded and still subject to powerful but subtle morality and ideological battles.

Coordination of remedial efforts in Africa remains a challenge as African leaders and institutions are yet to develop a continental strategy and program on HIV/AIDS. International assistance (bilateral and multilateral) remains focused on meeting donor needs, priorities and expectations.

African AIDS orphans are still on their own. By 2010, according to various estimates, up to 20 million AIDS orphans will live in Africa.

Women continue to bear the brunt of HIV/AIDS in Africa. In many heavily infected countries, girls between the ages of 15 and 19 are four times more likely than their male peers to be infected with HIV. Poverty, lack of viable economic opportunities, and draconian cultural practices continue to increase the vulnerability of African women to HIV infection.

Lack of international financial resources to fight HIV/AIDS in Africa continues to hamper local and national remedial efforts in Africa. The Global Fund to Fight AIDS, TB and Malaria is struggling to receive all promised monies from Western governments. The Fund's request for markedly increased resources from the West, especially the United States, is yet to receive a positive response.

Lack of transparency in government operations in Africa remains a silent but deadly obstacle to the mobilization of international resources against HIV/AIDS in Africa. It is critical for African leaders to remove any obstacle, perceived or real, that can hamper speedy remedial efforts against HIV/AIDS in the continent.

Hard Choices

To win the fight against HIV/AIDS in Africa, there are four unavoidable hard choices that must be made.

The first choice is to mobilize resources to provide anti-retroviral drugs to more than 4 million Africans that experts believe will immediately benefit from this treatment. The availability of antiretroviral drugs should occur simultaneously with the revamping of health systems in Africa. The United States and the rest of the G-8 nations have a special responsibility to make this happen because of historical and economic ties with Africa. Until HIV/AIDS becomes perceived as a chronic disease in Africa rather than a death sentence, most remedial efforts are unlikely to have much success.

The second choice is that HIV/AIDS remedial efforts in Africa should be decentralized or devolved to local communities where individuals infected and affected by HIV/AIDS live and die. The jury is still out on ongoing international remedial efforts, since it is not yet proven that these efforts so far are meeting the needs of individuals infected or affected by HIV/AIDS.

The third choice is that African governments must be held accountable for the prudent use of domestic, continental and international resources mobilized to fight HIV/AIDS in the continent. If the silent tug-of-war between rich nations and African governments continues on this issue, then the capacity to mobilize huge resources will be severely damaged.

Finally, it is crucial, as I have argued in my previous writings, that Africa leads this battle against HIV/AIDS in the continent. To lead this battle, Africa must have a common strategy on HIV/AIDS remedial efforts, and engage current and prospective international partners with clearly articulated policies and programs.

These are hard choices that will require a change in current practices and norms. However, these choices are necessary to fight the gravest development challenge to Africa's renewal and prosperity.

---

* Remarks made as the Moderator of the Panel on Updates on Africa on the Global Challenges of HIV/AIDS organized by the US Congress Human Rights Caucus, April 1, 2004

7

HIV/AIDS AS A SECURITY ISSUE *

(October 2001)

The terrorist attack on America killed about 3,000 people on September 11, 2001. The international community mourns the loss of thousands of innocent lives from more than 40 nations. A global coalition of nations led by America is fighting back against terrorism.

I am gratified that the Congressional Black Caucus, especially the Foreign Affairs Brain trust committee led by Congressman Donald Payne, organized this session on HIV/AIDS even as the resolve to fight terrorism is unwavering and the country is still in mourning. Please, join me in recognizing the long-term commitment to Africa's development by Congressman Donald Payne.

This session is important because every day, at least 15,000 individuals contract the HIV virus that causes AIDS, according to Helen Gayle of the Bill and Melinda Gates Foundation. More than 95 percent of daily infections are in developing countries and about 13,000 are in persons aged 15 to 49 years. In Africa, every day about 11,000 individuals contract HIV and nearly 7,000 die of AIDS.

According to the United Nations agency coordinating the response to the HIV/AIDS (UNAIDS), an estimated 36 million people are currently living with HIV. At the current rates of HIV infection, more than 100 million people worldwide will be living with HIV/AIDS by 2015. The toll of war in the 20th century stood at 33 million while 22 million people have already lost the battle for life to AIDS in the last twenty years of the 20th century. AIDS now kills ten times more people a year in Africa than war.

The epicenter of this dreaded epidemic is Sub-Saharan Africa. Seven African countries already have prevalence rates of 20 percent or more. By 2010, at least 20 million AIDS orphans will live in Africa. In Sub-Saharan Africa, AIDS may eventually kill one in four adults.

The security implication of unprecedented deaths from AIDS is enormous. According to the World Bank and UNAIDS, by the time infection rates reach 20 percent in a country, gains in health, longevity and infant mortality are wiped out. The projected situation in South Africa, Zambia, and Zimbabwe by the end of the decade readily comes to mind, with expected major reversals in health indicators, life expectancy and infant mortality rates.

AIDS prevalence of 20 percent or more also comes with security implications for countries struggling to overcome economic difficulties. At this prevalence rate, according to the International Crisis Group, food supply becomes tenuous, families struggle to maintain basic household needs and communities strain under economic losses. Young, unemployed people are more likely to adopt fatalist attitudes toward life. Social unrest, crime, and economic refugees surge.

Perhaps the greatest security threat of HIV/AIDS, especially in Sub-Saharan Africa, is that the best and brightest in the heavily infected countries are the first to contract HIV and likely die of AIDS. By 2005, according to Helen Gayle of the Bill and Melinda Gates Foundation and one of our speakers today, AIDS is expected to claim the lives of between 8 and 25 percent of current medical doctors in six countries of southern Africa. The political class in Africa is also under attack from AIDS as top government functionaries and parliamentarians have died of the disease. Top-flight business executives, journalists, and academics have been lost to AIDS.

The International Labor Organization predicts that AIDS deaths in many African countries would likely reduce the proportion of experienced workforce in critical sectors of the economy. As inexperienced colleagues replace these experienced workers, production costs, already high in Africa, will skyrocket with attendant continuing loss of international competitiveness. The AIDS crisis is already forcing some employers in Africa to train two or more workers for the same job as a safeguard against the real possibility of losing key employees to AIDS.

High rates of AIDS deaths are also likely to fracture the fragile democratic foundations of many African nations as the incidence grows in the powerful armies of African nations. Estimates from the World Bank, UNAIDS and the Economic Commission of Africa put HIV prevalence rates in the military of African nations from 10 to 50 percent. In many African nations, according to the International Crisis Group, the rate of infection among the military is as much as five times that of the civilian population. It is highly unlikely that the Military High Command will tolerate the specter of officers dying without access to lifesaving HIV medicines.

As we listen to the speakers, it is important to remember HIV/AIDS affects families, communities, governments, security agencies, and economic institutions. As the economic and social engine rooms of society - young and productive citizens - disappear or become incapacitated, African countries already wobbling from economic and political problems can implode from within.

HIV/AIDS is indeed a development emergency and a security threat to the prosperity of developing nations, especially African countries.

Invited Presentation at the US Congressional Black Caucus Foreign Affairs Brain trust, Capitol Hill, Washington, DC delivered in October 2001

PART II:

HIV/AIDS AND AFRICA'S RESPONSES

8

HIV/AIDS AND AFRICA: BACK TO THE DRAWING BOARD

(November 27, 2002)

After 21 years of dealing with the HIV/AIDS epidemic in Africa, it appears that Africa has now reached the crossroads. According to the United Nations agency coordinating the pandemic (UNAIDS) nearly 30 million Africans live with HIV/AIDS. More than 21 million Africans are dead of AIDS. At least, four African countries - Botswana, Lesotho, Swaziland and Zimbabwe - have more than 30 percent of their adult population living with HIV/AIDS. Only 30,000 Africans have access to lifesaving, available antiretroviral medicines. Despite these unfolding ugly scenarios, Africa is yet to mount or lead a credible fight against the number one developmental crisis in the continent.

On a "positive" note, African leaders are committed to spending 15 percent of their national budget on health care at the 2001 Abuja summit on HIV/AIDS. Many African countries have "completed" or at the "advanced stages" of completing national strategic plans against the epidemic. Many African leaders now "speak out" against the disease. Many African countries are now "streamlining" their HIV/AIDS remedial efforts in their anti-poverty strategies. African leaders are now fine tuning an ambitious development initiative known as New Partnership for Africa's Development (NEPAD). However, for a continent that is losing its most productive citizens on a daily basis and is dealing with a ballooning AIDS orphan problem, these "positives" are clearly not enough. Africa must go back to the drawing board and come up with a comprehensive strategy and operational mechanism to fight this deadly disease.

What are these HIV/AIDS Strategies and Operational Mechanisms?

The first important strategy is that Africa must stop looking outside the continent for leadership in the fight against HIV/AIDS. Charity must begin at home. I call on the leadership of the African Union, NEPAD, the UN Economic Commission for Africa (ECA), the African Development Bank, the civil society and professional groups to create an African body to fight AIDS in the continent. This African led and managed institution will be responsible for setting priorities for both for local and external funded activities; resolving lingering issues about access to care; overcoming infrastructure impediments; and, implementing information, education and communication (IEC) strategies. Today, in Africa, any external organization can decide which part of Africa it wants to assist in the fight against HIV/AIDS and the priorities for its assistance.

The second strategy is that HIV/AIDS must become an integral part of NEPAD. It is not possible to talk about Africa's renaissance or economic growth without a serious attention to the number one development priority of the continent. The third strategy is that Africa must mobilize its professionals in the continent and Western countries to fight this epidemic. The fourth strategy is for Africa to develop and implement a common approach to developmental assistance from the West. NEPAD is a good start but needs to demonstrate internal capacities and mobilization of resources, and also carry along all key stakeholders, including the civil society.

Regarding operational mechanisms, it is crucial for Africa to focus on two key issues: medical and health related aspects of HIV/AIDS, and the developmental consequences of HIV/AIDS. The medical and health related aspects of HIV/AIDS include a strong resolution to provide lifesaving drugs to Africans living with HIV/AIDS. Anything that stands in the way of this resolution must be tackled jointly by all African governments. In addition, African leaders must commit to reach every high risk African with a credible IEC message on how to prevent HIV transmission and how to avoid re-infecting other people if already living with the virus.

To deal with the developmental consequences of HIV/AIDS, African leaders should focus on accelerated food production, since nutrition is an important facet of the fight against the disease.

UNAIDS concluded that the current famine in Southern Africa is related to the ongoing HIV/AIDS epidemic in the region. Coupled with accelerated food production, African leaders should regard the reduction of agricultural subsidies by Western nations as one of their most important developmental strategies. According to the Chief Economist of the World Bank, the average subsidy to every cow in the European Union is now about US$2.50, higher than the daily incomes of Africans among whom more than 40 percent live on less than one dollar a day. To overcome widespread economic crisis, Africa must trade its way out of poverty.

Additionally, African leaders - in the interest of their own people and not because of pressures from donor nations - should focus relentlessly on improving the social and economic circumstances of their citizens. Poverty is at the nexus of the HIV/AIDS epidemic in Africa as individuals continue to take calculated behavioral risks in the daily struggle to fend for themselves and their families. Finally, the elimination or drastic reduction of Africa's unsustainable debt in a swap for accelerated expenditures in health care and social services is very crucial in the short term to create a breathing room for governments struggling to meet the basic needs of their citizens.

After years of living in Washington, DC, I know that nobody will help Africa unless it is ready to help itself. I am also aware that it is highly unlikely that the West will step up its developmental assistance to Africa if there are lingering doubts about the commitment of African governments. I am also aware that if Africa does not mobilize its resources - at home and abroad - in the fight against HIV/AIDS, developmental partners will continue to make obligatory gestures rather than substantial commitments. There is a growing donor fatigue about HIV/AIDS in the West, and advocates for greater commitment will receive a substantial boost if Africa gets its act together. Will Africa seize the opportunity to lead the world in the fight against HIV/AIDS? I hope so.

References

Chinua Akukwe (2002). "African-African American cooperation in the global fight against HIV/AIDS." Remarks at the US Secretary of State Open Forum. September 2002. Available at http://www.state.gov/s/p/of/proc/tr/13526pf.htm

Chinua Akukwe (2002). "HIV/AIDS in Africa: An integrated regional approach." *Africa Notes*, July/August 2002, pages 7-11. Institute for Africa's Development, Cornell University, Ithaca, NY.

UNAIDS (2002). *Report on the Global HIV/AIDS epidemic*. June 2002. Geneva: Author.

UNAIDS, World Health Organization (2002). *AIDS Epidemic Update*. December 2002. Geneva: Author.

United Nations General Assembly (2002). *Report of the Secretary-General on Progress towards Implementation of the Declaration of Commitment on HIV/AIDS*. Released August 12, 2002. A/57/227. New York: Author.

9

AFRICA AND NEPAD: WHAT ABOUT HIV/AIDS?

(April, 2002)

The African-conceived and led New Partnership for Africa's Development (NEPAD) is an ambitious attempt by African leaders to jumpstart development in the continent. However, NEPAD as currently articulated lacks a serious focus on the HIV/AIDS epidemic in Africa. As a vehicle for Africa's renaissance, based on indigenous initiatives and focused external support, NEPAD must be seen as a vehicle for tackling major impediments to the economic growth and political stability in Africa. The HIV/AIDS epidemic is unarguably the greatest threat to Africa's development at this point in time. I discuss why HIV/AIDS should be on the shortlist of any NEPAD strategic priorities.

Current Focus of NEPAD

NEPAD is touted as a "holistic, comprehensive integrated strategic framework for the socioeconomic development of Africa." NEPAD provides a "vision for Africa, a statement of the problems facing the continent and a program of action to resolve these problems..." The goals of NEPAD include (a) promoting accelerated growth and sustainable development, (b) eradicating widespread and severe poverty, and (c) halting the marginalization of Africa in the globalization process. Sectoral priorities of NEPAD include bridging the infrastructure gap in the continent; human resource development initiative (poverty reduction, higher education attainment levels, reversing brain drain, and health); agriculture; the environment; cultural issues, and science and technology.

As African leaders prepare to engage their G-8 counterparts during the June 2002 meeting in Canada, the current focus of NEPAD is on five areas of development:

1. Capacity building on peace and security.
2. Economic and corporate governance.
3. Infrastructure development.
4. Financial standards and the establishment of a Central Bank.
5. Agriculture and market access.

These focus areas of development in NEPAD are appropriate and deserve commendation. However, it is difficult to contemplate a serious attempt at jumpstarting development in Africa without urgent attention to HIV/AIDS, a condition that can negate not only the vision of NEPAD but also its goals, priorities, and current areas of focus. I briefly review the effect of HIV/AIDS on NEPAD's goals, priorities and current areas of focus.

HIV/AIDS and Goals of NEPAD

HIV/AIDS is a formidable foe of accelerated growth and sustainable development in Africa. According to the World Bank and UNAIDS, HIV/AIDS in the hardest hit countries of Africa is directly responsible for an annual loss of 0.5-1.2 percent of GDP. This is in a continent that must achieve a growth rate of 7 percent to meet the United Nations Millennium Development Goals (MDG) of halving poverty levels by 2015. By 2020, heavily infected countries may lose up to 20 percent of their GDP to AIDS. HIV/AIDS is also fingered as a major factor in the current life expectancy in Africa of 47 years instead of 62 years without AIDS.

HIV/AIDS is also a deadly opponent of any serious poverty alleviation effort in Africa, where at least four of every ten individuals live on less than $US1 a day. By picking off the most productive segments of the society, AIDS creates a cascade of poverty enhancing effects at family, community and national levels.

The World Health Organization's Macroeconomic Commission in its recent report estimates that regions that suffer truncated lives from early deaths and chronic disability stand to lose billions of US dollars a year. According to UNAIDS, in Botswana, where every third adult is living with HIV/AIDS, one quarter of households can expect to lose a breadwinner within 10 years, and per capita household income for the poorest quarter of households will fall by 13 percent. As breadwinners fall sick and die, household income dries up, food becomes increasingly scarce and/or rationed, children are pulled out of school, and poor families spend limited savings and household holdings on fruitless AIDS palliative treatment. Communities are deprived of their best-trained leaders, and nations suffer from the untimely deaths of their best bureaucrats, technocrats, doctors, nurses, teachers and other pro-fessionals. Public expenditure on healthcare will go up at a time of declining tax revenue from limited numbers of productive workers.

Africa's marginalization in the globalization process is exemplified, according to the World Bank, by its almost zero share of global manufactured goods, less than 2 percent of global trade, and its reliance on volatile commodity prices as sources of foreign exchange.

As a continent that exports mostly non-processed goods, Africa, in addition to the impediments of massive agricultural subsidies imposed by the West, must deal with its small domestic markets that are dependent on the HIV/AIDS ravaged tiny middle class. Business organizations in many parts of the AIDS hard-hit Southern Africa have to hire two or more persons for the same job, and are incurring heavy costs in absenteeism, insurance premiums and death benefits.

At least 28 percent of miners in South Africa are believed to live with HIV/AIDS. According to both the World Bank and UNAIDS, private investments are not likely to flow consistently to countries that are losing their best workers to AIDS, because of stagnating demand and high labor costs. Farmers are also at the receiving end of HIV/AIDS: the International Labor Organization, an arm of the UN, estimates that at least 7 million farm workers in Africa have died of AIDS, and millions more are still at risk. In addition, critical investments in soil enhancement and irrigation are drying up because of the epidemic, according to the UNAIDS.

HIV/AIDS and NEPAD Priorities

The HIV/AIDS epidemic in Africa put the searchlight on the poor healthcare infrastructure in many countries, including the hardest hit nations. The healthcare system in Africa, in decline for a long time, became inundated with the needs of individuals dying of AIDS. In some countries in Southern Africa, AIDS patients occupy more than 50 percent of all hospital beds. The inadequacies in transportation, energy, telecommunications and information management became glaring in the moral battle to extend lifesaving antiretroviral drugs to Africans living with HIV/AIDS, as opponents repeatedly cited these inadequacies.

Human resource development initiatives in Africa must deal with pervasive effects of HIV/AIDS as experienced workers die and younger workers remain at risk. As noted by UNAIDS, the loss of transfer of knowledge between more experienced workers and younger employees, and the higher recruitment cost of replacing sick and dying workers, can increase the workers' compensation budget of a typical manufacturing outfit by 10 percent or more in Africa. Far more important, the millions of young men and women that look healthy today and are potential beneficiaries of human resource initiatives may be living unknowingly with HIV that will manifest clinically in less than a decade.

The effect of HIV/AIDS on the environment is still unfolding. However, human beings, the best stewards of the environment in Africa, are already at risk of HIV/AIDS. The cultural ramifications of loosing generations of citizens to AIDS will likely be significant. However, one cherished cultural tradition in Africa, the extended family system, is already under strain from the unprecedented waves of AIDS orphans. Science and technology will also take a major hit as the likely elite users die of AIDS and technical workers fall sick.

HIV/AIDS and the Current Focus Areas of NEPAD

Peace and security in Africa may come under threat in Africa if the estimated high rates of HIV infection in the powerful African armies hold up. The World Bank, the UN Economic Commission for Africa and UNAIDS estimate that infective rates in the rank-and-file of national armies in Africa range between 10 and 50 percent. It is highly unlikely that military commanders will tolerate the specter of high death rates and lack of access to lifesaving drugs. The United States Institute of Peace and the International Crisis Group have provided compelling evidence of how conflicts, massive movements of people, displaced communities, and refugee status facilitate the transmission of HIV through rape, sexual coercion, and trading sex for survival.

Economic and corporate governance, infrastructure development, enthroning transparent financial standards, establishing a Central Bank, improving agriculture output, and increasing access to markets, domestic and abroad, depend on skilled and productive workforce in the public and private sectors. HIV/AIDS remains a formidable threat to the current and future workforce in Africa.

What to do

HIV/AIDS is a major impediment to the lofty goals and objectives of NEPAD. I believe that African leaders should immediately adopt HIV/AIDS remedial efforts as one of the focus areas of NEPAD, and set in motion a machinery to translate the Abuja 2001 declaration on HIV/AIDS into a working document for the forthcoming meeting with G-8 nations.

The HIV/AIDS working document should address critical issues such as access to antiretroviral drugs, culturally appropriate information, education and communication (IEC) campaigns, and mobilization of Africans everywhere to fight the epidemic. The working document should define the relationship between NEPAD and other players in international AIDS remedial efforts, and document the parameters of aid for development programs regarding HIV/AIDS (UNAIDS estimates that at least 80 percent of resources needed to fight AIDS in Africa will come from external sources). Additionally, the working document should set out specific parameters for accelerated debt relief in exchange for verifiable investments in HIV/AIDS remedial efforts, and for holding African governments accountable in national and local campaigns against the epidemic.

Finally, NEPAD should be an opportunity to develop a continental response to the HIV/AIDS epidemic as part of the new

African Union (AU). Although the NEPAD document alludes to the work of the Global Fund for AIDS, Malaria and Tuberculosis, UNAIDS, and other active players in the international arena, the HIV/AIDS epidemic has the capacity to neutralize the lofty aims of African leaders enshrined in the envisaged partnership for development. With 28 million Africans living with HIV/AIDS and more than 20 million already dead, the number one development emergency in Africa deserves priority attention in NEPAD, the touted vehicle for the continent's accelerated development.

10

HIV/AIDS IN AFRICA: LESSONS LEARNED*

With Ronald Dellums, Jack Kemp and Melvin Foote (December, 2001)

As we mark World AIDS Day and ponder the fate of 40 million people worldwide living with the disease, it is an opportune time to reflect on the lessons learnt so far in the ongoing remedial efforts in Africa, the epicenter of the AIDS epidemic. Although the international community is now sharply focused on the war against terror, we believe that international efforts to contain AIDS in Africa should be on course. It is important as part of continued international action against AIDS to review lessons from current remedial activities in Africa. Lessons learned today can serve as a guide for better strategies in the future.

Lessons Learned

A global response, led by the Western democracies, is needed in the fight against HIV/AIDS in Africa. Kofi Annan, the Secretary General of the United Nations, estimates that the fight against HIV/AIDS globally will require $7 billion to $10 billion per year. Resources needed to fight AIDS globally and in Africa require the active involvement and generous support of rich nations, including the United States. It is our belief that the war on terrorism should not preclude active and adequate support for HIV/AIDS remedial efforts in Africa. The Bush Administration and other Western leaders should continue their support for the fight against AIDS in Africa. The proposed Global Fund for HIV/AIDS, TB, and Malaria is an important instrument for action in Africa.

African governments are crucial in the battle against AIDS. We are happy to note that African nations have taken up the leadership challenge, especially after the April 2001 regional conference in Abuja, Nigeria. The United Nations identifies lack of leadership as the Achilles heel of any serious response to AIDS. African governments are now committed to significant and steady funding for HIV/AIDS programs.

Civil societies in the West and Africa are critical stakeholders. In the last few years, organizations in North America and Europe advocating for an effective constituency for Africa have demonstrated the capacity of powerful ideas and organizational skills to influence public policy regarding HIV/AIDS. African-based civil societies are also in the forefront for a just and equitable approach to remedial actions against the epidemic.

Treatment and prevention programs are needed simultaneously in anti-AIDS efforts. The United Nations agency coordinating the HIV/AIDS response (UNAIDS) estimates that nine out of every ten infected Africans are unaware of their status. Treatment options are now widely recognized as a powerful incentive for getting tested. Africans living with HIV/AIDS, like their counterparts in the West, should have access to lifesaving antiretroviral therapy. Additionally, in the absence of a vaccine and cure, the prevention of new HIV infection should be the gold standard of any serious remedial effort. As shown in this country, Europe, Senegal and Uganda, individuals can alter their behavior and reduce their risk status following a comprehensive, culturally appropriate information, education, and communication (IEC) campaign.

Poverty, tuberculosis and other sexually transmitted diseases create a fertile environment for HIV transmission. These conditions are endemic in Africa. As noted by UNAIDS, the epidemic feeds on existing social and economic problems in high-risk communities. Both TB and sexually transmitted diseases create ideal conditions for HIV transmission. Remedial action against HIV/AIDS in Africa will require concerted effort to curb the effects of these conditions.

Gender inequities in Africa represent a significant threat to AIDS remedial efforts. Africa is the only continent where more women are living with HIV/AIDS compared to men. African women should be front and center in the fight against HIV/AIDS.

68

African governments and civil society organizations should address gender inequities that inhibit the capacity of women in Africa to respond to HIV/AIDS at family, community, and national levels.

Public/private partnerships are needed to address the various ramifications of the epidemic. In Africa, the best and brightest are mostly affected by the epidemic, with serious economic and social consequences. In addition, many of the African nations with high rates of infection have limited resources. Business organizations in Africa now have to grapple with the insidious effects of AIDS. In the southern region of Africa, the most affected in the continent, businesses are now forced to hire two or more persons for the same job as a safeguard against AIDS. Public/private partnerships in Africa are now critical in designing and implementing IEC campaigns, improving access to anti-retroviral therapy for company employees and family members and sharing expertise in strategic planning and logistics as nations gear up their response to the epidemic.

AIDS orphans represent a major threat to the long-term survival of communities in Africa. The rising incidence of children who have lost their parents or mothers may become the ultimate legacy of the AIDS crisis in Africa. The United States Agency for International Development (USAID) estimates that by 2010, at least 40 million AIDS orphans will live in Africa if the present state of infection and death continues unabated. Unless specific and direct efforts are taken to safeguard these orphans, Africa may suffer enormous social, economic and cultural consequences as these children grow up without extended family support and care.

Steady advances in science have assisted remedial efforts. Advances in drug regimens are prolonging lives in the West. We look forward to a similar situation in Africa. The science of vaccine production is steadily improving. Findings from epidemiological and ethnographic studies are already influencing the design and implementation of IEC campaigns. There is a growing list of collaborative scientific relationships between Western based establishments and their African counterparts.

Yes, you and I can make a difference. The motto of this year's World AIDS Day is "I Care...Do You?" As noted by UNAIDS in its recent publication, *Together We Can*, individuals, communities, institutions, and governments can make a difference in the fight against HIV/AIDS. What is needed is a unity of purpose, clarity of mission, willingness to dialogue, pooling of resources and the capacity to mobilize for action. The fight against HIV/AIDS is likely to be won one person and one community at a time. Making a difference will also require identifying best practices and replicating them wherever necessary.

We are gratified with the growing involvement of today's young people in the design and implementation of HIV/AIDS policies and programs around the world. The active participation of young people is a positive sign that remedial actions against HIV/AIDS in Africa will likely continue until the threat of epidemic significantly abates.

For a disease that infects almost 600 people every hour world-wide and kills more than 60 children during the same time period, time indeed is of the essence. It is even more urgent in Africa where more than 28 million people live with HIV/AIDS. In Africa, we must channel our creative energies into action to save lives and secure future generations.

* Honorable Ron Dellums is the Chairman of the Constituency for Africa Washington, DC; former US Congressman, and; former Chairman of the US House of Representatives Armed Forces Committee;

Honorable Jack Kemp is the Vice Chairman of the Constituency for Africa; former Republican Vice Presidential Candidate; former US Secretary for Housing and Urban Development, and; former US Congressman;

Melvin Foote is the President/Chief Executive Officer of the Constituency for Africa, Washington, DC.

11

HIV/AIDS IN NIGERIA: AVERTING AN IMPENDING CATASTROPHE*

(September, 2000)

Nigeria, the "giant" of Africa, is currently at a crossroads. From the religious uprisings in the North to the ethnic conflicts in the South, the serious crime situation, and the Executive-Legislative brawl, Nigeria is always boiling. However, Nigeria may be stewing in a potentially devastating problem that is yet to attract the sustained attention of its elite and international well-wishers: the unfolding epidemic of HIV/AIDS.

According to the United Nations Agency on AIDS (UNAIDS); nearly 3 million Nigerians live with HIV or are dying of AIDS, a prevalence rate of 5 percent. In some urban centers, the prevalence is more than 15 percent among the adult population, and at least 20 percent among pregnant women. HIV/AIDS disproportionately affects future leaders of Nigeria: Nigerians aged 20 through 39 account for more than 70 percent of all infections. Nearly 85 percent of all HIV transmission occurs through heterosexual contact. Nigeria has one of the highest rates of HIV by unsafe blood transfusions (14 percent) in the world. Conservatively, UNAIDS estimates that 1.7 million Nigerians have died of AIDS, and more than 1.3 million children have been orphaned.

The Political, Social, Economic, Health Consequences of HIV/AIDS in Nigeria

At the present trend of infection, by the year 2020, 75 million Nigerians may live with the HIV virus. These infected Nigerians will live under a certain death sentence unless rapid strides are made in vaccine development and administration. For the millions of Nigerians living with HIV, and slowly dying from AIDS, their preoccupation is unlikely to revolve around the major national issues of today: Sharia; North versus South power shift; Executive versus Legislative fight for supremacy; ethnic struggles for control of natural and man-made resources; Military versus civilian control of government. Of course, these national issues are important for the corporate survival of Nigeria. However, the HIV/AIDS epidemic has the potential to disarm both the Sharia warriors and their antagonists, waste the political elites, rob these elites of their "supporters," decimate the military, and render mute the ethnic-based struggle for economic empowerment.

With one in five Africans a Nigerian, the road to an effective control of the HIV/AIDS pandemic in Africa leads through the rough and sometimes slippery political terrain of Nigeria. An explosion of HIV/AIDS will not only destabilize Nigeria but will have far reaching repercussions for the whole of Africa.

HIV/AIDS is an equal opportunity disease, without any respect for social class distinctions. It is also impervious to religious, ethnic or political beliefs, and thrives in conditions of sustained socioeconomic chaos as are presently evident in Nigeria. Any country that does not seriously address the future consequences of HIV/AIDS is sitting on a keg of gunpowder.

Nobody should underestimate the effect of HIV/AIDS on the economic, healthcare, political, and social stability of Nigeria. For example, the biggest threat to a stable political environment in Nigeria may not be the number of nocturnal meetings by top military officers. It is likely to be the specter of a rising incidence of HIV/AIDS in the Nigerian military. With a reported 10-15 percent infection rate, the Military High Command in Nigeria, or any country for that matter, is unlikely to tolerate high numbers of "untreated" AIDS soldiers and officers. Simply put, unchecked HIV/AIDS is a national security threat to Nigeria and its budding democracy. Additionally, a growing rate of infection in the public sector portends grave social and economic dangers. The International Labor Organization, an arm of the United Nations, estimates that the labor force of Nigeria will decline by between 3 and 9 percent by 2020 if the present trend of the infection continues.

The surviving Nigeria labor force will be younger, less educated, and will have limited experience in governance. Since most civil servants in Nigeria are the major breadwinners of their immediate and extended families, the fragile socioeconomic situation in Nigeria may implode. As shown by studies in other African countries, HIV/AIDS can lead to the untimely deaths of critically needed teachers, medical personnel, engineers, top-level bureaucrats, and farmers. We may never know the true cause of death of prominent Nigerians that died after a "brief" illness. However, as noted by Professor Olikoye Ransome-Kuti, the former Minister of Health, most families of AIDS patients will strenuously object to a listing of AIDS in the death certificate of their dead relatives.

High rates of HIV/AIDS often translate into higher operating costs for business entities. Businesses will spend more money on sick and low productive workers, curtail their expansion plans, and look for areas or countries with low-cost burdens. Consequently, the poor business environment in Nigeria will get worse no matter the macroeconomic policies of the government because of sick workers and unhealthy potential customers.

HIV/AIDS is also likely to exacerbate the grinding poverty in Nigeria, pushing it higher than the current levels of more than 60 percent. Steady advances in girl education may falter as girl-orphans are less likely to continue schooling. The unprecedented wave of orphans will strain the extended family system, and eventually lead to these orphans fending for themselves. Most of these orphans will end up as social miscreants, prostitutes, political or economic enforcers, and hardened criminals.

The comatose healthcare system in Nigeria will go into a state of suspended animation because of HIV/AIDS. Most AIDS patients suffer repeated bouts of infection from opportunistic diseases. These patients require varying lengths of expensive hospitalization, occupying scarce hospital beds and consuming dwindling healthcare resources. In a country that rarely spends more than 3 percent of its national budget on health care, and operates mostly poorly equipped hospitals and health centers, it is highly unlikely that the health system in Nigeria can withstand the strain of caring for terminally ill AIDS patients with multiple opportunistic infections. The collapse of the Nigeria healthcare system is a distinct possibility as it reels from years of limited funding, the exodus of experienced medical personnel to Western and Middle East countries, and the high cost of private care.

The Response of the Nigerian Government

This is not the place to exhaustively address the reported response of the Government to the HIV/AIDS epidemic. However, I will present a brief overview. The Nigerian government reportedly set aside $1million for AIDS control effort during this year. This is clearly too little for the task at hand. On a happier note, President Obasanjo has spoken publicly on HIV/AIDS, appointed a national policy council headed by himself, and another technical advisory committee headed by an experienced AIDS researcher, Professor Ibironke Akinsete. The Federal Government is planning an international conference on HIV/AIDS in April 2001 in Abuja. The Government reportedly took delivery of testing equipment from the European Union and recently completed a national "Action Plan." Various state governments such as Lagos and Nasarawa reportedly have active HIV/AIDS prevention programs. President Clinton during his recent visit made specific financial commitments to Nigeria's HIV/AIDS program.

However, the Federal Ministry of Health is in the news because of its apparent protracted struggle with Dr Jeremiah Abalaka * who claims to have developed a vaccine against the HIV virus. This matter is before the Courts and the National Assembly. Suffice to say that it is important to re-echo the wise admonition of Nelson Mandela during the closing ceremony of the 13th HIV/AIDS conference in Durban, South Africa: Every African should focus on how his/her action will affect those individuals living with HIV and AIDS, and those at risk of contracting the infection.

Implementing a Response to the HIV/AIDS Epidemic in Nigeria

With one in five Africans a Nigerian, the road to an effective control of the HIV/AIDS pandemic in Africa leads through the rough and sometimes slippery political terrain of Nigeria. An explosion of HIV/AIDS will not only destabilize Nigeria but will have far reaching repercussions for the whole of Africa. Fortunately, the basic elements of successful HIV/AIDS programs are known. The World Bank estimates that a credible national HIV/AIDS program will likely cost 1.5-2.0 percent of GDP.

A credible national response to HIV/AIDS in Nigeria should have the following strategic thrusts:

(1) President Obasanjo should declare HIV/AIDS a national security threat to Nigeria and should mobilize appropriate financial, technical, and political resources to checkmate the spread of the epidemic.

(2) Nigeria should link its crusade for debt relief with a clearly articulated HIV/AIDS program. Nigeria is groaning under an international debt estimated at $31 billion, of which $17 billion is owed to the Paris Club of creditor countries, and the rest to the London Club of mostly commercial banks. This debt accounts for nearly 75 percent of Nigeria's annual GDP, a major headache for the leadership of the country where the average citizen earns $320 per year. Nigeria spends about $1.5 billion or 4 percent of its GDP on debt servicing, three times its budgetary allocation for education, and nine times its outlay for healthcare.

(3) Nigeria should develop and implement a national Strategic and Action Plan for combating HIV/AIDS. This national strategy should involve individuals living with HIV/AIDS, civil society, and community representatives in all phases of policy formulation and implementation. It should also be multi-sectoral, comprehensive, and appropriate for the medical and development ramifications of the disease.

(4) Nigeria should provide clinical care to HIV/AIDS patients. Nigerian health authorities can benefit from the experiences of Brazil and Thailand, and the ongoing struggle by South Africa to procure cheaper generic versions of lifesaving antiretroviral drugs.

(5) Nigeria should implement credible information, education, and communication (IEC) campaigns to prevent new infections, modify risky behavior, and ensure that infected individuals do not transmit the virus. Nigerians should engage in a national dialogue on the risk factors of HIV transmission, how to avoid the infection, and how to manage the infection. Religious entities, non govern-

mental organizations, and community-based welfare or impro-vement unions are the key elements of a credible IEC program.

(6) Nigeria should mobilize the private sector to participate in local, state, and national HIV/AIDS programs. The private sector is a critical partner in developing and implementing work site programs, reducing unemployment and poverty, and assisting in the logistics of moving drugs and equipment.

(7) Nigeria should promote research in vaccine development, qualitative studies, and safer drug regimens. Nigeria should be at the forefront of vaccine development for the African strains of HIV, and should work closely with Nigerian experts at home and abroad in this regard. Every claim for the "cure" of HIV/AIDS should be promptly and properly investigated.

(8) Nigeria should embark on a massive resuscitation of its healthcare infrastructure. This is an area that can benefit very quickly from a debt repayment "swap" with investments in health-care.

Nigeria, like every other powerful nation, will continue to face multiple problems. However, the HIV/AIDS epidemic is a remorse-less, opportunistic foe that can tear Nigeria apart. Nigeria's fragile polity burdened by deep ethnic jingoism, religious tensions, and internecine struggle for national resources will be frayed at the edges by unchecked rampage of HIV/AIDS. This disease will likely drain scarce national financial resources and may lead to irreversible social upheavals.

---

* Not much has been heard on the Abalakka issue in recent years.

76

12

HIV/AIDS IN AFRICA: SOUTH AFRICA'S LEADERSHIP IS CRUCIAL

(December 2003)

The recent announcement that South Africa's government will roll out a comprehensive anti-retroviral treatment program by the end of September 2003 is a major step in the right direction for the estimated 5 million South Africans living with HIV/AIDS. It is also a giant step forward for the more than half a million South Africans who need immediate access to antiretroviral therapy. A comprehensive and effective treatment plan for South Africa is also welcome news to South African families that dread the death of a loved one from AIDS: Every day, at least 600 South Africans die of AIDS associated illnesses.

That the first ever National AIDS conference only took place in August 2003 in a country with the highest known case load of HIV/AIDS is a testament to the titanic struggle between the government and civil society organizations in South Africa on the best way forward on HIV/AIDS, the Achilles heel of the country's otherwise rosy economic future. Various reports from the National AIDS conference suggest that South Africa is now entering the "death" phase of the epidemic, with devastating implications for the national economy, the workforce, and the powerful private sector. One of the reports by the Human Sciences Research Council of South Africa (HRSC) indicated that in a recent survey, 16 percent of 2,000 surveyed health workers were HIV positive, with at least 20 percent of those aged 20 to 35, living with the virus.

Although South Africans will benefit immediately from their government's decision on access to AIDS treatment, the widest implication for the new AIDS policy in South Africa will be for the continent of Africa. As the economic juggernaut of Africa, a pre-eminent military power, and an oasis of reasonable democratic traditions, South Africa is a giant in the continent. Today in Africa, South Africa and Nigeria are without exception, the two most powerful and influential nations in Africa. A lot is expected of South Africa as Nigeria grapples with its myriad of problems. For Africa to tackle its number one development emergency, HIV/AIDS, South Africa must not only be on board, but also provide vigorous leadership.

A popular question is why South Africa becomes gun shy when it comes to a vigorous response against HIV/AIDS. Many analysts have noted the influential role South Africa played in the transformation of the increasingly ineffectual Organization of African Unity into a promising African Union. South Africa's role as the gentle but firm guiding hand in the formulation of the Africa's recovery plan, NEPAD, is well known. The proposed AIDS comprehensive treatment program may be seen as an attempt by South Africa to reassert its leadership role in the continent.

However, as with other policy announcements in Africa, the devil is in the details, and saints can only be crowned with evidence of vigorous implementation and sustainability of laudable programs, even for a known and deadly killer such AIDS. South Africa must not only roll out an effective treatment program, it must also expand such services at an accelerated rate to reach those that are clinically qualified for treatment. The current estimate is that out of 500,000 South Africans that can benefit from antiretroviral therapy, only 21,000 are on lifesaving therapy. Medical charities serve more than 95 percent of all those on antiretroviral therapy in South Africa. South Africa, in addition to a comprehensive treatment program, must improve its information, education and information (IEC) campaigns against HIV infection. This will require regular IEC messages on HIV prevention from President Thabo Mbeki.

At the continental level, South Africa should ensure that the African Union and NEPAD not only talk about HIV/AIDS but also devote substantial resources in a continent-wide fight against the disease. If Africa should have a home-grown economic recovery plan, why should it not have an African-oriented AIDS remedial effort? An effective African oriented AIDS remedial effort would go beyond conference declarations and resolutions to specific issues such as cross sharing of expertise and resources across borders, strategic priorities on resource sourcing and mobilization, and the role of Africans in the Diaspora.

South Africa's continental leadership role is also crucial in current efforts to allow poor nations to obtain cheaper versions of AIDS drugs using the mandates of the World Trade Organization. In addition, South Africa's flourishing research institutions have a lot to offer many African nations that are still developing their capacities for quality scientific research. South Africa, with its well-developed private sector and a sophisticated civil society, is also in a position to offer continental leadership on an effective tripartite approach - public, private, civil society - to AIDS remedial efforts. In the area of governance, now emerging as a major handicap in AIDS remedial efforts in Africa, democratic traditions and institutions in South Africa, despite occasional hiccoughs, appear robust and stable, and could provide pointers to other African countries.

I look forward to South Africa's robust leadership of AIDS remedial efforts in Africa. As a member of the Constituency for Africa's delegation to NEPAD and South Africa in early 2003, I observed first hand the no-nonsense approach to leadership by South Africa's leaders. During the delegation's lengthy audience with the Deputy President of South Africa, Jacob Zuma, he spoke eloquently on how HIV/AIDS had become a major problem for his country. Now, it appears that the government of South Africa is ready to lead its people out of mortal danger from AIDS.

A strong resolve and necessary action against HIV/AIDS in South Africa will not only affect its citizens but will also have far reaching implications for the continent of Africa. The Economic Commission of Africa in its latest report on Africa estimates that HIV/AIDS, on the average, reduces Africa's GDP growth by 0.5-2.6 percent a year, dealing mortal blows to the expected annual 7 percent GDP growth needed by Africa to meet the 2015 UN Millennium Development Goals. South Africa, as the economic engine room of Africa and as one of the "big two" politically in

Africa (Nigeria is the other country), cannot afford to be missing in action in the fight against the gravest threat to Africa's renaissance.

13

HIV/AIDS, SOUTH AFRICA AND DEMOCRACY

(April, 2004)

The African National Congress (ANC) and Thabo Mbeki's government won a resounding mandate from South African voters in April 2004. With this renewed mandate, Thabo Mbeki will serve his second and final term as president until 2009. Despite the anticipated margin of victory by the ANC, a visitor to South Africa in the last few weeks would have noticed how Thabo Mbeki and his senior colleagues in ANC campaigned vigorously throughout the country. A major reason for the vigorous campaign was to repair a breach of trust between the government and South Africans over the country's HIV/AIDS policies and programs.

That the government of South Africa miscalculated in the war against HIV/AIDS is not news. What is really newsworthy is that for the first time, the issue of HIV/AIDS forced a popular government and a popular political party to backtrack and engage in major reversals of public policy. From initial skeptical public postulations on AIDS etiology and specific clinical treatment protocols, the government of South Africa read the mood of its citizens on the epidemic and acted by rolling out the most comprehensive and ambitious treatment plan in Africa. Furthermore, the government faced the unenviable task of re-introducing itself to hard-core supporters who have been at the receiving end of the HIV/AIDS epidemic. The treatment program is at its infancy but the government's commitment to HIV/AIDS remedial efforts is no longer in doubt.

The gravest challenge to South Africa's future in the next two decades is likely to be the fallout of HIV/AIDS. As the country with the largest concentration of individuals living with HIV/AIDS, at least 5 million, South Africa faces a future that will herald untimely deaths of its most productive citizens, a potential spiraling cost of private enterprise in the country due to sickness and death of skilled workers, and a devastating epidemic that targets the poor in South Africa. According to various estimates by multilateral agencies and South Africa research institutions, the HIV/AIDS epidemic in South Africa is going to take its toll even if the government does every thing right. Thus, any delay in executing decisive remedial efforts, is potentially dangerous.

The April 2004 election reaffirmed the faith of South Africans in ANC and its government led by Thabo Mbeki. On HIV/AIDS, South Africans gave the government the benefit of the doubt. By the next election in 2009, South Africans will have enough evidence to assess its government's commitment on HIV/AIDS.

For other African nations preparing for elections in the next few years that have a growing number of individuals living with HIV/AIDS, the die is cast. These countries may wish to learn from the recent predicament of the ruling party in South Africa. Nigeria, Zambia and Kenya should take particular note of the South Africa's situation since they have growing rates of HIV/AIDS, limited government remedial efforts, high rates of poverty, and a polity that is far from stable.

Forthcoming elections for post-conflict Democratic Republic of Congo, Liberia and Sierra Leone may also revolve around the fate of infected returnees and those families that bore the atrocities of the conflict, including rape. These countries in the next few years will get to know the full extent of their HIV/AIDS epidemic, the socioeconomic impact, and the potential degrading of the law and security apparatus.

As politicians and policy makers become increasingly aware that HIV/AIDS is a major development emergency and a potential political deal breaker between citizens and their governments, the future of remedial efforts looks bright in Africa. Some may argue that South Africa's government respects the majesty of the ballot box and may have fought scared in a credible election to reclaim a mandate that could not have gone elsewhere, at least for now. However, for governments that have less respect for the ballot, they must be prepared to deal with the consequences of an enraged citizenry hobbled by grinding poverty, incensed by growing suffering and death from AIDS, and exasperated by lack-luster response from their leaders on remedial efforts.

If the most powerful government in Africa, controlling the most powerful economy and arguably the best army, had to work hard to regain the trust of its citizens on HIV/AIDS, then less powerful African governments must be wary. HIV/AIDS once crossed the Rubicon from health care into the development arena. HIV/AIDS has made another move, and is now firmly ensconced in the political arena in Africa.

A report on the eve of the election in South Africa by the Governance and AIDS Program (GAP) of the Institute for Democracy in South Africa suggested that HIV/AIDS is already threatening democracy in the country since most eligible voters are within the same age range of individuals most affected by the epidemic. GAP even suggests that the integrity of the next South Africa election in 2009 may be compromised by high rates of HIV/AIDS among prospective voters and electoral staff. If millions of individuals become sick or are dying of AIDS in future elections, then, who will campaign, vote or oversee the elections? Without doubt, HIV/AIDS in Africa is now out of the shadows, forever ending two decades of deafening silence in the continent.

Selected Bibliography

1. Akukwe, C. (2003). "HIV/AIDS in Africa: South Africa's Leadership is Crucial." *The Perspective,* Atlanta, GA. http://www.theperspec tive.org/aids_southafrica.html.

2. UN Integrated Regional Information Network (IRIN) (April 9, 2004). "South Africa: Special Report on a Decade of Democracy-HIV/AIDS." Johannesburg. Available at http://www.irinnews.org/AIDSreport.asp&Reportpercent20ID=3252. This is a comprehensive policy, program, research and chronological update of the HIV/AIDS situation in South Africa.

3. UN Integrated Regional Information Network (IRIN) (April 9, 2004). "South Africa: HIV/AIDS Threatens to Undermine Democracy."

Johannesburg. Available at http://www.irinnews.org/AIDSreport.asp& Reportpercent20ID=3251.

4. Haacker, M. (2003). "Providing Health Care to HIV Patients in Southern Africa." IMF Discussion Paper. PDP/01/3. Washington, DC.

5. Topozis, D. (2003). *Addressing the Impact of HIV/AIDS on Ministries of Agriculture: Focus on Eastern and Southern Africa.* Joint FAO/UNAIDS Publication, Rome.

6. South Africa Business Coalition on HIV/AIDS (SABCOHA), South Africa Bureau for Economic Research (2004). *The Economic Impact of HIV/AIDS on Business in South Africa, 2003.* Johannesburg, South Africa.

7. South Africa Consulate General, New York (2003). "Cabinet's Decision on the Operational Plan for Comprehensive Care and Treatment of People Living with HIV/AIDS and AIDS. Questions and Answers." Available at www.southafricanewyork.net/consul ate/sppeches/hivaids19nov2003.htm

8. South Africa Bureau for Economic Research (2001). *The Macro-Economic Impact of HIV/AIDS in South Africa.* No. 10. Available at http://www.ber.sun.ac.za/downloads/2003/aids/aidsma cro_sep2001.pdf

PART III:

TUBERCULOSIS AND MALARIA: FORGOTTEN DISEASES?

14

MALARIA AND TUBERCULOSIS: FORGOTTEN DISEASES*

(April 2004)

I have written extensively in the print and electronic media about the unfolding HIV/AIDS epidemic in Africa and the far-reaching development implications of a lack-luster remedial effort. In writing or making presentations on HIV/AIDS in Africa, I am not unmindful of the deadly consequences of two "forgotten diseases" in Africa and other developing regions, Malaria and Tuberculosis (TB). These two diseases are not just endemic in most countries with high prevalence of HIV, but also account for extensive personal suffering and death. Malaria and TB appear to be "forgotten" because they are widely known in endemic areas and often believed to be under "control" with available drugs. In addition, the high death toll associated with both diseases is not common knowledge.

What do we know about Malaria and TB?

Malaria is one of the most common diseases in the world and throughout the tropical climates of the world. According to the World Health Organization (WHO), about 40 percent of the global population, mostly in the poorest countries, are at risk of contracting Malaria. The disease is a protozoa (plasmodium) infection, mostly transmitted from person to person by female *Anopheles* mosquito bites. *Plasmodium Falciparum* is the most common cause of Malaria in Africa. Malaria infects between 300 and 500 million people every year. The WHO estimates that every year, Malaria accounts for at least one million deaths. .

Malaria is particularly dangerous in Africa. The disease is responsible for 900,000 deaths in Africa every year. Every 30 seconds, an African child dies of Malaria. Every day, at least 3,000 Africans die of Malaria. At least 20 percent of all under-five child deaths in Africa are attributable to Malaria. Every year, 500,000 African children develop cerebral Malaria, a dangerous form of the disease with high mortality. Survivors may be left with severe neurological damage.

Pregnant women in Africa are also at grave risk from Malaria. According to the WHO, the disease is a major cause of morbidity and mortality during pregnancy in Africa. Malaria illness during pregnancy can cause spontaneous abortions, neonatal deaths (within the first 28 days of life) and low birth weight. In endemic areas in Africa, Malaria by *Plasmodium Falciparum* is responsible for 10,000 maternal deaths. In addition, Malaria accounts for 8-14 percent of all low birth weight babies and 3-8 percent of all infant deaths in endemic areas of Africa.

Tuberculosis (TB) is equally deadly. According to the WHO and the Global Fund to Fight HIV/AIDS, TB and Malaria (the Global Fund), at least one-third of all humanity harbors the bacillus that causes TB. Under certain conditions, these individuals can transform from latent TB to active status, with the capacity to infect others. The predominant mode of person-to-person transmission is through inhalation of bacilli released during coughing by infected persons. At least, 8 million individuals become sick with TB every year. TB is also a major killer: about 2 million people die of the disease every year. At least 250,000 of these deaths are children. The WHO estimates that by 2020, one billion people will contract TB and 35 million will die.

Africa is also at the receiving end of TB. At least 1.5 million TB cases are diagnosed every year in Africa. TB is also engaged in a deadly tango dance with HIV in Africa. Both the United Nations Agency coordinating the Response to HIV/AIDS (UNAIDS) and the WHO estimate that one third of all individuals living with HIV will eventually contract TB. In addition, TB is a leading killer of people with AIDS.

Economic Cost of Malaria and TB

In addition to the morbidity and mortality attributable to Malaria and TB, the economic cost of these two conditions is staggering. The WHO estimates that Africa loses US$12 billion a year because of Malaria. In a typical endemic area in Africa, 40 percent of public health expenditure, 30-50 percent of inpatient admissions, and up to 50 percent of outpatient visits is linked to Malaria. The economic effect of Malaria is so severe that endemic countries can lose up to 1.3 percent of their GDP every year to the disease.

The economic cost of TB is also high. According to the WHO, TB reduces the income of the poorest nations in the world by US$12 billion a year. An intricate web exists between TB and poverty. Countries with GNP of less than US$2,995 (low-income countries) account for 90 percent of all TB cases and deaths, according to the WHO. TB deaths are most common among the economically active segment of the population, at ages 15 through 54.

Despite the alarming morbidity, mortality and economic costs associated with Malaria and TB, the true extent of the disease is still unknown, especially at household levels. The effect of an episode of Malaria or TB on a breadwinner of a poor family is probably incalculable. This breadwinner, during an episode of Malaria or TB, may not work, may lose an existing job or may expend meager savings in seeking medical attention. This can further mire this poor family into deeper levels of poverty. In addition to the high economic cost of Malaria and TB, the development challenges are equally formidable.

Development Challenges of Malaria and TB

Known prevalence and incidence may be the tip of the iceberg; the grim statistics on Malaria and TB may not represent the full extent of these diseases. It is no secret that in a typical African setting, the treatment of suspected Malaria episodes often starts with self medication, then consultation with untrained medicine dealers, before winding up in a clinic or hospital. For TB, the WHO estimates that current diagnosed cases worldwide represent less than one-third of all potential cases, even in the West.

Both Malaria and TB have a wide geographical spread. They are endemic over a wide geographical area, and this has major implications for travel and control measures. Malaria is endemic in 45 African countries. It is also endemic in 21 countries in the

Western Hemisphere. The disease is common in East Mediterranean and South East Asia. TB is endemic in Africa. However, the highest burden of TB is in South East Asia. TB is also common in the Western Hemisphere. Its incidence is increasing in Eastern Europe, in parallel to an explosive upsurge in HIV infections. In this era of globalization, travel within and between countries and continents, it is a major challenge to provide effective remedial efforts against diseases that are common in wide geographical areas.

Intricate relationship with endemic poverty: Both diseases are common in poverty-stricken areas. Remedial efforts may hinge on the effectiveness of anti-poverty strategies.

Resistance to available drugs aggravates the problem. Both diseases have high susceptibility to multi-drug resistance against cheap but effective medicines. In addition, no new drugs for Malaria or TB has been developed or commercialized in the last two decades. According to the WHO, resistance to chloroquine, a popular antimalaria drug, is high in Africa, especially in Southern and Eastern Africa. Resistance to second line drugs (sulfadozine-pyrimethamine) is growing in Africa. To complicate issues, fake antimalarial drugs are commonly available, especially in West and Central Africa. The WHO recommends that all countries with resistance of 15 percent or more for frontline antimalarial drugs should switch to a combination therapy, especially Artemisin-based combination therapies (ACTs). However, ACTs at a cost of around US$2 per treatment is 10-20 times as expensive as chloroquine. For poor African countries, switching to ACTs is a tall order unless international financing is available. The Global Fund is providing assistance to some African countries in this regard.

Wars and instability facilitate transmission. Both Malaria and TB thrive under unstable conditions where individuals live in close quarters and in large numbers, exposed to the elements, and are focusing on personal survival rather than preventive measures against known diseases.

Breakdown of primary health systems worsens the problem. This is a sad situation since Malaria and TB, at early stages, are eminently treatable in community clinics and primary health care centers. However, in Africa, primary health care centers are often ineffective due to limited or inconsistent funding, poorly trained or motivated staff, and the inability to provide continuity of care. Community-based preventive systems against Malaria and TB are lacking in most endemic areas in Africa.

Poor application of control measures can be dangerous: both Malaria and TB require completion of full course of prescribed drug regime for effective clinical care. This is a challenge in many resource-poor communities. Preventive efforts are also at risk in these communities as high-risk individuals are often focused on day-by-day economic, mental and emotional survival. For example, an early sign of a Malaria attack may not dissuade a poor farmer from tending to his or her invaluable crops, a critical source of cash for family needs. This poor farmer sooner rather than later may be rushed to a health facility with a more serious form of malaria.

In addition, Malaria and TB thrive in malnourished individuals. Malnutrition compromises the immune system, creating a perfect condition for Malaria and TB infection and complications. Malnutrition is common in Africa, especially among children less than five years of age.

Women are at risk of contracting or dying of Malaria and TB. Pregnant women are in grave danger from Malaria, especially in Africa. Women are less likely than men to be tested for TB in Africa.

Despite the formidable development challenges of Malaria and TB, there are emerging silver linings in organized remedial efforts. I briefly discuss these silver linings.

Silver Linings

First, the emergence of multi-sectoral, global alliances dedicated to comprehensive remedial efforts against specific diseases is changing the strategies for communicable disease control and prevention. These alliances represent an active collaborative effort between governments, the private sector and the civil society. Each alliance identifies specific impediments to effective remedial efforts against specific diseases, and mobilizes financial and technical resources toward overcoming the obstacle. Global alliances have emerged over the last few years against malaria, TB, and HIV/AIDS. The Global Fund against AIDS, TB and Malaria is a major example of a global resolve to fight specific diseases, singly or in combination.

Second, the availability of concentrated funds to address specific diseases is another silver lining. A major player in providing concentrated funding against specific diseases is the Gates Foundation. By deploying vast amounts of targeted resources, the Gates Foundation is galvanizing policy, program, research and logistic effort against specific diseases worldwide. Some of these efforts include vaccine development programs against HIV, and immunization of millions of children against preventable childhood diseases.

Third, the politicization of communicable disease control and prevention has revolutionized remedial efforts. Heads of state and governments now routinely meet at the United Nations or in regional meetings to discuss communicable disease control and prevention strategies.

Finally, there are ongoing attempts to harmonize donor programs on communicable diseases in recipient countries or regions. The United States' $15 billion, five-year initiative against HIV/AIDS, TB and Malaria in 12 African and two Caribbean countries is a typical example.

For Malaria and TB, the most important global development in the past few years has been the emergence of the Roll Back Malaria initiative and the STOP TB Partnership. The Roll Back Malaria Initiative (RBM) emerged from the meeting of 44 Heads of State and Government from Malaria-affected countries in Africa in Abuja, Nigeria four years ago. RBM is focused on (a) improving access to timely Malaria treatment for at least 60 percent of infected individuals, (b) protecting 60 percent of all individuals and families at risk of Malaria through insecticide-treated mosquito nets, and, (c) assuring that at least 60 percent of pregnant women in endemic areas have access to intermittent preventive treatment against Malaria.

The STOP TB Partnership is focused on implementation of WHO's recommended Directly Observed Therapy Short Course (DOTS). DOTS operates on five basic strategies: strong political commitment in endemic countries; comprehensive microscopy service/back up for directly observed clinical care; assured drug supply of the highest quality; coordinated surveillance and monitoring systems; and use of effective therapies under direct daily observation. According to the WHO, 69 percent of world population live in geographical areas with access to DOTS.

What are the next steps in consolidating remedial efforts against Malaria and TB? I will focus on Africa.

Next Steps for Remedial Efforts in Africa

First, integrate Malaria and TB control and treatment into HIV/AIDS strategies in Africa. The Global Fund against AIDS, TB, and Malaria should be a rallying point for this effort. Every African country, especially those with endemic levels of HIV/AIDS, TB, and Malaria should develop a coordinated strategy against these diseases.

Second, the integration of control and treatment of HIV/AIDS, Malaria and TB should be replicated in regional and continental institutions in Africa. For example, the Economic Community of West African States (ECOWAS) should have an integrated strategy. The African Union should also have an integrated strategy.

Third, all bilateral and multilateral development partners active in Africa should re-align their strategies to incorporate joint HIV/AIDS, Malaria and TB remedial efforts.

Finally, Africa needs to revamp or establish community-based systems of clinical and preventive care. A community-based system of care that serves as the anchor for internationally directed remedial effort will provide timely assistance to individuals and families infected or affected by Malaria or TB.

Selected Bibliography

1. World Health Organization (2004). *Global Tuberculosis Control - Surveillance, Planning, Financing*. WHO/HTM/TB/2004.331. Geneva, Switzerland: Author. This is the latest, most comprehensive report on the global TB situation worldwide. Available at http://www. who.int/tb/publications/global_report/2004/en

2. World Health Organization (2004). *Guidelines for Malaria Control Recommended by RBM Department, WHO*. January. Geneva: Author. This is the latest guideline regarding Malaria control and prevention. Available at http://www.rbm.who.int/cmc_upload/0/0 00/017/113/who_recommended.htm. The RBM initiative has many

fact sheets and documents available for review at http://www.r bm.who.int/ including *The Economic Cost of Malaria* and *Malaria in Africa*. As part of World Malaria Day 2004, the WHO issued press release on malaria available at http://www.who.int/mediacenter/ releases/2004/pr-29/en.

3. Global Fund Against AIDS, TB and Malaria (2004). *The Global Tuberculosis Epidemic*. Geneva. This is a very good summary of the epidemic, and the social and economic implications. Available at http://www.theglobalfund.org/en/fighting/tuberculosis

4. World Bank (2004). *Communicable Diseases*. Washington, DC: Author. This is a summary of the effects of communicable diseases, including HIV/AIDS, TB and Malaria in Africa. Available at www.worldbank.org

5. Gates Foundation (2004). Information on its grant-funded program and recipients available at http://www.gatesfoundation.org

---

* *Excerpts from Continuing Medical Education (CME) Lecture delivered at the International Health and Travel Medicine Seminar organized by the Association of Scientists and Physicians of African Descent (ASPAD), Washington, DC, April 2004*

15

INTEGRATING TUBERCULOSIS AND MALARIA CONTROL PROGRAMS INTO HIV/AIDS REMEDIAL EFFORTS

(November, 2005)

As shown in the previous article on whether TB and Malaria are now forgotten diseases, the point is made that these two conditions are significant health issues in Africa. Together, with HIV/AIDS, TB and Malaria are priority health issues in most countries in Sub-Saharan Africa. For many poor rural communities and urban slums, death and illness from Malaria is a more important source of immediate concern that HIV/AIDS. Stigma associated with TB remains a formidable obstacle to effective preventive and treatment programs.

The co-infective status between HIV and TB in Africa as noted in the previous article is a major source of concern for clinicians and policy makers in the continent. In the Southern region of Africa, HIV and TB co-infections are now forcing governments to revamp their TB surveillance, control and treatment programs. The morbidity and mortality associated with Malaria in many regions of Africa is also gradually leading to a situation whereby domestic and international assistance programs are integrating anti-malarial remedial efforts with that of HIV/AIDS and TB.

The successful takeoff of the Global Fund against AIDS, TB and Malaria (The Global Fund) is also forcing various national coordinating mechanisms in recipient countries to integrate control and treatment efforts. The Africa Development Bank recently adopted a new communicable diseases guideline that recognized the primacy of HIV/AIDS, TB and Malaria as "priority diseases" for its financial and operational attention throughout the continent. I had served as the technical resource for the Bank in developing the new communicable diseases guideline. This new strategy by the African Development Bank is very significant since the institution is a major funding organization in Africa for health facilities, health care services and training programs for health workers.

To integrate TB and Malaria control efforts with HIV/AIDS remedial efforts, certain critical decisions need to be made at the highest levels of government and African-based institutions. First, national and institutional health strategies and policies should mandate such integration. Second, the integration should be mainstreamed in all programs and services at all levels of government and operational activities of African-based institutions.

Third, the economic impact of HIV/AIDS, TB and Malaria need to occupy prominence in economic planning and forecasting.

Fourth, the private sector needs to become major players in national and continental efforts to integrate HIV/AIDS, TB and Malaria remedial efforts. Experiences from the contribution of the private sector in HIV/AIDS remedial effort show that the business community can become major partners if show the effect of health conditions on the morale and contribution of their workforce.

Finally, community-based health systems and services should become the ultimate showcase of successfully integrated HIV/AIDS, TB and Malaria programming. Target communities and at-risk individuals should experience the benefits of integrated service delivery.

PART IV:

AIDS AND THE RESPONSE OF INTERNATIONAL ORGANIZATIONS

16

HIV/AIDS AND THE WORLD OF WORK: POLICY ADVOCACY ISSUES*

(September, 2004)

1. The role of the World of Work in HIV/AIDS remedial efforts is now well recognized thanks to the efforts of the International Labor Organization (ILO). The ILO HIV/AIDS program in three years is now a major strategic, policy and programmatic force in global efforts to stem the tide of HIV epidemic. Dr Franklyn Lisk, the Director of the program, and Honorable Assane Diop, the Executive Director for Social Protection, ILO, deserve special commendation for their work in the last three years.

2. The ILO program on HIV/AIDS and the World of Work is based on a tripartite arrangement of employees, employers, and governments. The tripartite framework of the ILO and its HIV/AIDS program provides a useful vehicle for mobilizing resources in poor countries. In many resource-poor regions such as Africa, the government is a major source of livelihood for most citizens. The private sector is also important, especially in countries that are the location of conglomerates such as South Africa and Nigeria. The gold mines of South Africa and oil fields of Nigeria are important testing grounds for the ILO's tripartite framework in AIDS remedial efforts.

3. It is important to closely observe the ongoing efforts to roll out a nationwide antiretroviral program in South Africa. I believe that the tripartite framework will be severely tested in South Africa for three main reasons: (A) The high prevalence and incidence rates of HIV in South Africa; (B) The significant influence of conglomerates in the national economy of South Africa, and; (C) The role of sophisticated trade unions that brought Apartheid to its

knees. In recent years, a fourth element, the academic community, especially policy-oriented institutions, have joined in organized efforts to improve HIV preventive programs and provide access to life enhancing therapy in South Africa.

4. For the Western countries, in this case the United States, the situation is radically different from that of resource-poor countries. The push for strong government response to HIV/AIDS came mostly from individuals and families living with HIV/AIDS. Then, the struggle moved to urban America where minority-based organizations and individuals living with the disease pushed both local and state governments to take action. At the national level, the US Congressional Black Caucus played a key role in getting the Clinton Administration to take a stronger stance on domestic AIDS remedial efforts.

5. Regarding advocacy efforts in the United States for Africa, the epicenter of the epidemic, African-focused or oriented organizations such as the Constituency for Africa and AFRICARE led the initial response. The Constituency for Africa (CFA) organized scores of high profile Town Hall meetings that brought together key stakeholders across urban and rural centers of the country. CFA, like most of the Africa-focused organizations, although located in urban areas, had extensive grassroots contacts with small town and rural based advocacy organizations and faith-based entities.

6. To champion AIDS remedial efforts in Africa, US based organizations focused on four strategies: (A) Fact-based policy reviews of intervention options and strategies; (B) Developing and sustaining relationships with members of the US Congressional Black Caucus; (C) Establishing mutually agreeable partnerships with organizations that are active in domestic HIV/AIDS remedial efforts and community-based development programs, and; (D) Forging relationships with academia, think tanks and research institutions on the science and strategies of remedial efforts.

7. In the United States, the role of the UN system in HIV/AIDS advocacy efforts is still evolving. The high profile given to HIV/AIDS by the Secretary General, Kofi Annan, has raised the visibility of the UN and its potential role in mobilizing public and private sector resources in America.

8. As we move into what I call the "financing" phase of HIV/AIDS worldwide, it is important to emphasize the tripartite framework championed by the ILO. This approach should combine the science of AIDS remedial efforts with the tough moral choices that policy makers in rich nations must face in the fight against this disease. Why should a man with four small children die in South Africa of AIDS when his counterpart in United States can manage his condition with lifesaving drugs?

9. As the private sector becomes increasingly visible and effective in the fight against HIV/AIDS, it is important to get business leaders to buy into the tripartite framework. This framework should be partnership-based rather than adversarial. It is also important to emphasize "what works" to business leaders. The impact of intervention programs should continue to receive appropriate attention. It is also important to emphasize process and impact indicators since they are crucial to winning new converts in decision-making positions in both the public and the private sector.

10. A major lesson I have learnt as a Board Member of the Constituency for Africa is that policy makers are willing to pay attention and act swiftly if advocacy is fact-based and respectful of contrary opinions and strategies. In the World of Work and HIV/AIDS program, we should focus on fact-based advocacy, partnership building, stakeholder comparative advantages, and maximization of scarce resources. The ILO and other UN agencies have a unique role as neutral arbiters to provide leadership in this process.

Finally, the role of resource poor countries in HIV/AIDS remedial efforts in their own countries is crucial. It is important for each country to be seen as seriously addressing the epidemic, even with meager resources. Each country should mobilize its stakeholders, ensure fairness and equity in the distribution of national resources, and make transparency in national affairs a priority. No country should allow a situation where concerns about its public accountability system or governance should be an inhibiting factor in internationally directed HIV/AIDS remedial efforts.

*Remarks at the Technical Briefing on HIV/AIDS and the World of Work at the UN General Assembly High Level Meeting on HIV/AIDS, September 22, 2003, United Nations Headquarters, New York)

17

HIV/AIDS GLOBAL TRUST FUND: A PROPOSED ORGANIZATIONAL STRUCTURE

Commentary, with Melvin Foote *
(July, 2001)

In an earlier article, we argued for an efficient and equitable governance structure for the proposed HIV/AIDS Global Trust Fund. As the G-8 nations meet in Genoa, Italy to finalize or possibly launch the Trust Fund, we believe that it is crucial for the donor nations to develop a sustainable partnership with recipient nations based on mutual respect and understanding. The Trust Fund offers the rare opportunity to develop and nurture a global development agenda that eschews the failed master-servant relationships of the past.

The World Bank in its March 2001 report on foreign aid programs in 10 selected African countries concluded that donor-imposed conditions are doomed to fail without the active partici-pation of the recipient nations in the design and implementation of such programs. The organizational structure of the proposed Trust Fund should reflect the perspectives of the key stakeholders in the global effort to stop AIDS in Africa and other parts of the world. It should also send reassuring signals to the taxpayers in the donor nations and the target populations in AIDS ravaged communities that the programs of the Trust Fund will reflect the identified priorities of proposed project areas. In addition, a balanced organizational structure would obviate the need for conditionalities and the subsequent remote control of the Trust Fund operations.

Proposed Organizational Structure

Vision Statement: To aggressively prevent new HIV infections and to provide comprehensive clinical treatment and social support for persons living with HIV or AIDS and other chosen health conditions. The Trust Fund will implement grant-funded programs.

Mission: (A) To reduce the incidence of HIV infection and other chosen health conditions such as TB and malaria.

(B) To provide ethically acceptable clinical treatment to persons living with HIV/AIDS and other chosen health conditions.

© To provide social support to individuals and communities ravaged by HIV/AIDS and other chosen health conditions.

(D) To provide and distribute effective HIV vaccine to high-risk populations as soon as practicable.

Board of Trustees: We propose a 34-member board of trustees, the highest decision making body of the Trust Fund. The Board of Trustees should provide strategic leadership to the Trust Fund. The Board will approve requests for grant-funded programs after careful reviews and deliberations. In addition, the Board will appoint the staff of the Global Fund secretariat, and supervise their activities. The Board of Trustees will comprise proven men and women in various disciplines with experience in public, private, and civil society governance issues. We propose that they serve for an initial period of three years, renewable for another three years. We recommend that the Board should meet every three months or more frequently depending on the circumstances. The composition of the Board should be as follows:

(1) One member from each of the G-8 nations (8 members), hereinafter referred to as the North;

(2) One member from each of the following developing regions, hereinafter referred to as the South: North Africa, Southern Africa, Western Africa, Eastern Africa, Central Africa, Asia, Latin America, and the Caribbean (8 members).

(3) Representatives of civil society, two from the North and two from the South (4 members).

(4) Representatives of persons living with HIV or AIDS, two from the North and two from the South (4 members).

(5) Representatives of the Foundations/Philanthropies, two from the North and two from the South (4 members).

(6) Representatives of the Private Sector, two from the North and two from the South (4 members). The representatives from the South should not be affiliated with Western conglomerates.

(7) The United Nations system (two seats to be determined by the UN Secretary General, and possibly rotated regularly to avoid turf battles between the various UN agencies).

The Chair of the Board of Trustees should come from the G-8 nations and the Vice Chair from the recipient nations. We recommend the following committees for the Board of Trustees: the Finance Committee to be headed by a representative of the South; the Technical Committee to deal with the professional issues of HIV/AIDS and other chosen health conditions; the Logistics committee to work on infrastructure and the movement of goods and services; and the Training committee to focus on clinical training programs, volunteer training, and community mobilization issues.

International Advisory Board

This Board will provide intellectual leadership to the Trust Fund. It will serve as a forum for sounding out complex issues confronting the Trust Fund. We propose a 20-member Board with a non-renewable term of three years. We feel that the Trust Fund should not become an avenue for the creation of an elitist class of "world class experts." Opportunities should be given to other professionals to participate in the activities of the Trust Fund. The Board should include experts in medicine, public health and development. The Board should comprise eight members from the G-8 nations, eight members from the recipient nations, and four members appointed on special merit. We propose that the Chair of the Board should come from the South and the Vice Chair from the North.

The Secretariat of the Global Trust Fund

In line with Kofi Annan's call, we support a "small" secretariat of dedicated and dynamic men and women that will implement the programs of the Trust Fund, and develop sustainable partnerships with other players in international development. We recommend a five-year term for the executive officers of the Trust Fund, with a rare renewable second term. We believe that the leadership of the Trust Fund should be "fresh," energetic and responsive to new ideas and opportunities.

The Executive Officers of the Trust Fund should be:

(1) The Director-General/CEO of the Global Trust Fund. This individual should be an expert on both HIV/AIDS and development. We recommend a representative of the South for this position, preferably from Africa, the epicenter of the pandemic. The Director General's office will likely include a small core support staff such as a Chief of Staff, a special assistant, a board liaison officer, a public relations officer, and an executive assistant.

(2) The Deputy Director General/Chief Operating Officer, to manage the day-to-day activities of the Fund. We recommend a representative of the North for this position. The Deputy Director-General staff will likely include a senior operations officer, a senior protocol officer, a senior human resources officer, and an executive assistant.

(3) The Executive Director, Finance to manage the fiduciary functions of the secretariat. We recommend a representative of the North for this position. This officer will likely be complemented by a senior financial officer dealing with financial policies and regulations; a senior financial officer to deal with disbursements, grants management, conferences, travel expenses, and training expenditures; and a senior financial officer for special duties and exigencies.

(4) The Executive Director, Logistics. This could be a military or NGO veteran with extensive experience in forward logistics, supply side management, and infrastructure development. This officer will probably require a senior logistics officer, a senior infrastructure officer, and an appraisal officer.

(5) The Executive Director, Technical Services to provide leadership on HIV/AIDS and other chosen health conditions. We recommend a representative from the South for this position. This position will likely require a senior clinical officer, a senior preventive officer, and a senior grant management officer.

(6) The Executive Director, Training to provide support for the training programs undertaken by the Fund. The support staff will likely include experts in information, education, and communication (IEC), volunteer training, community mobilization, and clinical training.

(7) The Inspector General, to provide internal and external audit and ethics oversight. We recommend a person from the South for this position to provide a balance to the Executive Director, Finance from the North. Support staff will likely include a senior audit officer (internal operations), senior audit officer (external operations), and a senior inspector, ethics.

Operations at Country Level

We do not recommend the creation of new structures in the recipient nations. The Trust Fund leadership should work with the UN country teams, host governments, the civil society and the private sector to implement delivery channels that meet the needs of the target population.

The TB infrastructure, primary care networks, and community-based development programs of developing should be the initial delivery mechanism for the Trust Fund.

Technical Relationships

We recommend that the Trust Fund should establish working technical relationships with various specialized UN agencies, think tanks, the organized private sector, and non government organizations. In Africa, the UN Economic Commission for Africa and the new and improved African Union (we hope) are crucial technical partners in the quest to marshal an effective continental response against HIV/AIDS and other health conditions deserving special attention.

The Emperor Must Wear Clothes

To avoid the proverbial specter of the emperor without clothes, we strongly urge that the leadership of the Trust Fund must run an open, transparent, ethical, and accessible program. In the fight against AIDS, we cannot afford an organization that is answerable to a select few, accessible to a privileged group of "experts," and responsive to the whims and caprices of faceless pressure groups. In view of the urgency of the task at hand, the Trust Fund must operate with a sole focus - providing relief to the millions of men, women, and children living with HIV/AIDS or chosen health conditions or at the risk of contracting new infections.

---

* Note: The initial structure of the Global Fund Against AIDS, TB and Malaria basically reflected the proposed organizational structure in this article. Till date, the Global Fund structure basically reflects issues discussed in this article.

18

HIV/AIDS IN AFRICA: WTO'S DECLARATION ON PUBLIC HEALTH IS A STEP IN THE RIGHT DIRECTION

With Melvin Foote
(November, 2001)

The ministerial conference of the World Trade Organization (WTO) ended in Doha, Qatar with a declaration on urgent global social, economic, and trade issues. However, a major stumbling block to pre-Doha consultations was the dispute over the WTO Agreement on Trade-Related Aspects of Intellectual Property Rights (TRIPS Agreement) and public health, especially as it relates to the raging epidemics of HIV/AIDS, Tuberculosis and Malaria. Africa is the epicenter of the HIV/AIDS epidemic with more than 25 million people living with the disease and at least 17 million people already dead.

We are pleased that wise heads prevailed in Doha with the separate declaration on the TRIPS agreement and public health. We are particularly gratified with the declaration that the "TRIPS Agreement does not and should not prevent Members from taking measures to safeguard public health." The ability of independent nations to protect the public health of their citizens and to facilitate access to essential medicines and goods should not be in dispute in the evolving ethos of globalization.

We are particularly pleased with Section 5, item C of the declaration that expressly states that "Each Member has the right to determine what constitutes a national emergency or other circum-stances of extreme emergency, it being understood that public health crises, including those relating to HIV/AIDS, Tuber-culosis, malaria and other epidemics, can represent a national emergency or circumstances of extreme urgency." Africa with its endemic health problems should benefit maximally from this declaration as it confronts the scourge of HIV/AIDS and other infectious diseases.

The civil society groups in both developed and developing nations that worked diligently on TRIPS and public health deserve special commendation. They have shown that it is possible to reshape international public policy by sophisticated intellectual and organizational tactics. The subsequent negotiations and rounds of trade talks call for continued vigilance and participation of civil society groups.

We look forward to greater cooperation and understanding between developed and developing nations regarding TRIPS and public health. The cost of inaction is substantial in Africa. According to Peter Piot, the Executive Director of the UN agency for HIV/AIDS, a 15-year-old teenager in South Africa or Zambia faces a lifetime risk of HIV infection and death from AIDS of over 50 percent without urgent remedial action. The war in Sierra Leone left 12,000 children without families while AIDS has already orphaned five times that number. By 2010, South Africa, the economic powerhouse of Africa (40 percent of the region's economic output), will likely face a real gross domestic product 17 percent lower than it would have been without AIDS. By 2010, 40 million AIDS orphans may live in Africa. The list goes on and on.

Finally, we believe that equitable and effective access to public health in Africa will require greater spirit of cooperation and action by the following key stakeholders: African governments; Western democracies, including the United States; research and generic pharmaceutical companies; multilateral agencies; and civil society organizations. Time is of the essence.

Selected References

World Trade Organization. *Ministerial Declaration*. Ministerial Conference, Fourth Session, Doha, 9-14 November 2001. WT/MIN (01)/DEC/W/1, November 14, 2001. (O1-5769).

World Trade Organization. *Declaration on the TRIPS Agreement and Public Health*. Ministerial Conference, Fourth Session, Doha, 9-

14 November 2001. WT/MIN (01)/DEC/W/2, November 14, 2001. (O1-5770).

Peter Piot (UNAIDS Executive Director). "AIDS and Human Security." Statement at the United Nations University, Tokyo, Japan, October 2, 2001.

Chinua Akukwe and Melvin Foote. "HIV/AIDS in Africa: Time to Stop the Killing Fields." *Foreign Policy in Focus Journal*, Vol. 6, No. 15, May 2001 (http://www.fpif.org).

PART V:

AIDS IN AFRICA AND THE
RESPONSIBILITIES OF THE WEST

19

HIV/AIDS IN AFRICA: WHAT WILL IT TAKE FOR THE WEST TO ACT?

With Melvin Foote
(April, 2001)

Imagine the reaction of the developed nations on the grim news that every American that resides in the states of Texas and Tennessee will die before the end of this decade from a deadly disease or that 80 percent of Canadians live with this fatal condition.

Can we imagine the international outcry if nearly 50% of British or French citizens lived with this deadly disease. Equally appalling would be the news that nearly one third of the German population or one fifth of Japanese citizens live under a death sentence from a preventable disease.

The developed nations would be up in arms to defeat this mortal enemy.

The resolve to fight would even be stronger with the news that the disease has already claimed 17 million lives. Panic would set in if it was revealed that 90 percent of all infected individuals are unaware of their status and may unwittingly transmit the infection to other people.

As implausible as the above scenario may seem, this is the situation in Africa where more than 25 million individuals live with the HIV virus that causes the fatal disease known as Aids.

According to the February 2001 report of the United Nations secretary general Kofi Annan, although Africa represents 10% of the global population, it is the home to 70 percent of adults and 80 percent of children living with HIV infection.

In 16 African countries, one tenth of the adult population aged 15 to 49, are infected with HIV. In the southern region of Africa, one in four women aged 20 to 29 live with the HIV virus. By the end of this decade these individuals will die of AIDS. Africa accounts for three-quarters of the nearly 22 million dead of AIDS since the epidemic began.

The dead, mostly young men and women left the care of their small children to grand parents and relatives living in poverty. By 2010, 20 million Aids orphans, children less than 15 years, will live in Africa.

According to the World Bank, within 15 years an unchecked AIDS epidemic in Africa will shrink its economy by 25 percent. This is in a continent where about half of its people live on US$0.65 a day.

Ominously, the United Nations estimates that 90 percent of infected Africans are unaware of their status. Africans at risk of HIV transmission are unlikely to come forward for testing and counselling as long as anti-HIV lifesaving drugs are out of reach. Less than one-tenth of one percent of the 25 million infected Africans have access to the lifesaving drugs that are readily available to Americans and the citizens of other Western countries. These drugs have changed AIDS from a fatal to feared but manageable disease in the West.

It is indeed puzzling that the unfolding AIDS tragedy in Africa is not attracting the same kind of outrage, concern or response that will occur if entire Western nations, states or cities face uncertain futures from a deadly disease. Instead, it appears that the developed nations are looking for excuses not to act decisively.

For instance, the major pharmaceutical companies have focused on enforcing patent rights rather than facilitating access to lifesaving anti-HIV drugs, the recent spate of announced price cuts notwithstanding. Europe is in frenzy over foot-and-mouth disease. America is burdened by struggles over tax cuts. The International Partnership Against AIDS in Africa (IPAA), a grand public/private/civil society partnership organized by the United Nations to address the epidemic in Africa, is headquartered in Geneva, Switzerland.

It is like having NATO commanders prevent or manage wars in Europe from an outpost in the Kalahari Desert. It appears that there are no shortages of AIDS conferences, consultations, and technical visits by various multilateral agencies.

Wealthy industrialized nations (G7) continue to wink at the massive external debts of impoverished African countries. The annual debt repayment schedules are so punishing that African nations such as Nigeria and Kenya spend more money on debt repayments than on education and healthcare combined.

Compounding the problem of international inattention and amnesia is the role of African leaders. The wars, killings, repressive policies, corruption, and economic woes continue unabated in many African countries.

Some African leaders would rather plunge their impoverished countries into chaos than leave office after constitutionally mandated terms.

Many African leaders are at "war" over minerals and barren pieces of land when the greatest war is unfolding in their midst. AIDS is the real war in Africa since it is now responsible for more deaths in the continent than all military wars combined in the last 50 years.

It is time for the developed nations to intervene forcefully to end the AIDS genocide in Africa. An African contracts HIV every 25 seconds.

Every day, nearly 7 000 African families bury a loved one who died of AIDS. At least 17 million Africans are already dead. How many more will die before we act?

History is not likely to remember the first decade of this century as the period of technological innovations, tax cuts or foot-and-mouth disease.

History will likely focus on what kind of people and their leaders would allow 25 million people to die needlessly from a disease that is not only controllable with available drugs but also amenable to intensive, albeit expensive information, education and communication campaigns.

20

HIV/AIDS: THE LOOMING FUNDING CRISIS

(July, 2005)

Three major recent events signal that financial support for international remedial efforts against HIV/AIDS may be facing an uncertain future.

First, UNAIDS in a report released in June 2005 projected a looming funding gap of US$18 billion for HIV/AIDS in developing nations between 2005 and 2007. The funding gap, according to UNAIDS, can scuttle ongoing strategies for access to comprehensive prevention programs against HIV transmission. It would also jeopardize the aim of providing antiretroviral treatment (ART) to 75 percent of individuals clinically qualified to receive these medicines in 2008 (about 6.6 million individuals). A funding shortfall between now and 2007 would also slow down the progress made in providing social and healthcare support for AIDS orphans and other vulnerable children affected by the pandemic. Critical programming costs and urgent training needs for health personnel would also suffer, according to UNAIDS, if the projected funding shortfall becomes a reality. Currently, none of the major donor countries, including the United States, have stepped forward on how to end the looming funding gap identified by UNAIDS.

Second, the Global Fund to fight AIDS, Tuberculosis and Malaria (The Global Fund) has already identified a funding gap of US$700 million for 2005 alone. In addition, the Global Fund estimates that it needs additional funding pledges from donor countries of about US$2.9 billion in 2006 and US$3.3 billion in 2007 to continue its cycle of replenishing successful country-based programs and supporting new grantees. In 2004, the Global Fund accounted for 20 percent of all HIV/AIDS funding worldwide. These funding gaps have the potential to undermine an invaluable by-product of the Global Fund mechanism: the belief by poor countries that they can plan ahead knowing that accepted proposals will get financial support and approved projects will get funded throughout the project cycle. It is instructive to note that the 2005 G-8 communiqué on the Global Fund only pledges to "meet the financing needs for HIV/AIDS, including through the replenishment this year of the Global Fund to fight AIDS, TB and Malaria."

Third, it appears unlikely that the World Health Organization (WHO) and its collaborating partners will succeed in the goal to provide 3 million people dying of AIDS with anti-retroviral treatment by 2005 in resource-poor countries ("3 by 5"). As of June 2005, the WHO estimates that about 1 million qualified individuals are now on ART as a result of the "3 by 5" program. It is important to note that the WHO estimates that 6.5 million individuals worldwide need urgent anti-retroviral therapy, immediately. In Africa, despite the tripling of individuals on antiretroviral therapy since WHO launched the "3 by 5" program 18 months ago, nearly 90 percent of those in need do not have access to ART.

In view of the major funding gaps in international HIV/AIDS remedial efforts, what are the prospects for additional funds in the next two years?

Prospects for Additional HIV/AIDS Funds

The prospects appear mixed. The declaration by G-8 leaders at their 2005 summit in Scotland to provide funds for "universal access" to anti-retroviral therapy by 2010 for those in need is a very significant positive development. The political leaders of the richest nations on earth are now on record as making a definite political commitment to end the current dichotomy of access to ART in developed and developing nations. The implication of the declaration is that G-8 leaders will increase financial and technical resources to meet the 2010 timeline.

The commitment of G-8 nations to fully meet the financial obligations of the Global Fund for 2005 is also encouraging. However, these commitments should be counterbalanced with somber news: every day, every week, every month and every year, fathers, mothers, sons and daughters who are clinically qualified for ART will die without immediate assistance to readily available medicines. The cost of avoidable delays in mobilizing and utilizing resources in the fight against HIV/AIDS is very finite for millions of individuals in need of ART: they will die.

The situation is especially bleak for Africans dying of AIDS. For the 4.2 million Africans currently in need of ART, the G-8 pledge of universal access to treatment by 2010 will be academic since most of them would have lost the fight against AIDS. Delays in providing a comprehensive HIV preventive program can only mean additional cohorts of new infected individuals and affected families.

Another important development is that a looming war appears in the horizon between donor and recipient countries on governance reforms. The 2005 G-8 communiqué is the most specific documentation of rich nations resolve to hold recipient countries accountable for verifiable progress in governance and anti-corruption measures. It is likely that G-8 nations will not redeem their pledges of additional financial assistance to recipient countries deemed lacking in governance.

On the other hand, recipient countries are likely to chafe against overt and subtle pressures from donor countries on yardsticks for governance, especially stamping out corrupt practices. Recipient countries will cite the need to let the judicial system take its course once public officials are indicted for corrupt practices rather than being stampeded to politically solve corruption cases. The next few years may witness heightened tensions as G-8 and other rich nations aggressively pursue governance reforms in recipient countries as a condition for increased development assistance.

Thus, a situation may arise within the next few years whereby disagreements on governance between donor and recipient countries may hold up the disbursement of urgently needed financial and technical resources for HIV/AIDS remedial efforts. The irony is that HIV/AIDS target populations in recipient countries will bear the brunt of the disagreements over governance reforms. Future attempts by donor countries to "reward" good economic or political "performers" in recipient countries will also consign

HIV/AIDS positive citizens of non-favored nations to second class status and avoidable suffering and death.

What can be done to end the looming funding crisis for HIV/AIDS remedial efforts in resource-challenged environments?

Ending a Potential HIV/AIDS Funding Crisis

First, the G-8 and other rich nations should pledge to meet all verified HIV/AIDS funding shortfalls between now and 2010 in order to satisfy two important remedial goals: providing comprehensive preventive services to individuals at risk of contracting HIV, and providing universal access to treatment for all individuals clinically qualified to receive anti-retroviral therapy.

A pledge sooner rather than later by G-8 nations will have the benefit of allowing bilateral and multilateral agencies and recipient governments to plan ahead knowing that all legitimate HIV/AIDS program needs will be met. An immediate pledge by G-8 and other rich nations to meet all legitimate shortfalls in HIV/AIDS funding between now and 2010 would also set in motion a comprehensive process for verifying HIV/AIDS funding needs so that politicians and policy makers can make a more convincing case to their tax payers. A funding pledge by G-8 and other rich nations would also force recipient countries to set up verifiable indicators of governance since donor countries have already pledged to support legitimate funding needs. G-8 nations should honor their pledges as and when due.

Second, all poor countries with more than 5 percent HIV prevalence should have one hundred percent debt cancellation with the savings invested in verifiable programs. The G-8 nations deserve commendation for the cancellation of the debt of 18 poor countries. However, in the fight against HIV/AIDS, AIDS hit poor countries should not service foreign debts when their citizens are dying because of lack of access to available medicines. The cancellation of the debt burden of AIDS-hit poor countries will also force recipient country governments to accelerate their governance reforms and take concrete steps to combat corruption. In addition, the civil society of these countries will become active watchdogs of their government and policy makers.

Third, it is now critical to resolve donor concerns about governance in recipient countries. It is no secret that donor countries are growing increasingly frustrated with lack of progress on governance issues in recipient countries. Misappropriation of funds, difficulties with organizing legitimate elections, inability to secure lives and property, lack of independent judiciary, marginalization of minorities, limited capacities to enforce contracts and monopolization of political power are major concerns of donor countries. The relatively weak standing of national civil society organizations and human rights watchdogs are also complicating governance reforms in many recipient countries.

It is now time for donor and recipient countries to establish PRINCIPLES OF GOVERNANCE with verifiable indicators that are public knowledge to tax payers in donor and recipient countries. These principles should apply to all governments and there should be no sacred cows in recipient countries. Donors should also not play favorites and should not provide sanctuary for ill-gotten gains from recipient countries. For recipient countries, it is critical for opposition parties, professional associations and the civil society to play a verifiable watchdog role on HIV/AIDS remedial programs.

Finally, it is critical to reform HIV/AIDS remedial efforts with a principal focus on how to meet the needs of individuals and families infected and affected by HIV/AIDS. In the last five years, steady progress has been made on mainstreaming HIV/AIDS in the political, economic and social arena. The rich nations have set a timeline (2010) for universal access to ART. Recipient countries are moving more into population-based democracy and making gains in governance. Debt cancellation as a weapon in the fight against HIV/AIDS is now widely accepted.

However, what has failed so far is efforts to fund a way to make a difference in the lives of individuals and families batting with HIV/AIDS. Very few domestic or international HIV/AIDS remedial programs can provide a verifiable answer to a basic question: How many individuals living with HIV/AIDS received direct benefits as a result of the remedial effort? How many families affected by the sufferings of a loved one living with HIV/AIDS received direct benefits from the remedial effort?

Today, while AIDS remedial efforts continue to mature and become more sophisticated, target populations in resource-poor countries remain outside their sphere of influence. There is a danger that AIDS bureaucracy, public and private, worldwide may become more important than the needs of target populations. A lack of impact on the target population may lead to an increasing emphasis on process indicators as barometers of HIV/AIDS remedial efforts. The lack of significant, sustained impact on the target population may lead to celebration of modest program success for a pandemic that kills more than 2 million people every year. For example, in Africa, is it correct to celebrate the fact that only 500,000 people out 4.7 million qualified individuals (about 11 percent) are on ART?

For a pandemic that had been around for more than two decades, the lack of impact of remedial efforts at individual and family level is remarkable. The needs of the target population should now assume primacy after more than two decades of the pandemic.

Every AIDS agency should focus on how its actions or inactions affect the individual or family dealing with HIV/AIDS. Every measurable indicator should include evidence of how specific action will impact individuals and families dealing with the pandemic. Future funding estimates and projections should show verifiable evidence of how past remedial efforts impacted individuals living with HIV/AIDS and their families.

Conclusion

A funding crisis looms in HIV/AIDS remedial efforts in resource-poor countries. UNAIDS estimates a funding shortfall of US$18 billion between now and 2007. A funding shortfall would have devastating consequences on steady gains made in HIV preventive programs and access to lifesaving, antiretroviral therapy. G-8 and other rich nations should step forward and ensure that HIV/AIDS remedial efforts remain fully funded. Recipient nations should ensure that concerns about governance and corruption become a thing of the past. HIV/AIDS remains a deadly pandemic, killing more than 2 million people every year. Individuals and families infected and affected by HIV/AIDS should become the cornerstone of future HIV/AIDS remedial efforts.

21

HIV/AIDS IN AFRICA: UNAVOIDABLE FOREIGN POLICY PRIORITY FOR THE BUSH ADMINISTRATION

(February, 2001)

President George W. Bush is settling down to his responsibilities as the leader of the United States and the "free world". As the leader of the sole super power, the President's moves and actions send signals across the globe. Nowhere is the power of the American presidency felt more than in the foreign policy arena. For example, despite the landslide election of Ariel Sharon in the Prime Minister elections of Israel, America will continue to "guide" Israel and the Palestinians to the negotiating table. The NATO alliance will continue to rely on American influence and Military might. The Koreans will sustain their fragile peace under the watchful gaze of American soldiers. The President, the Secretary of State, Colin Powell, and his foreign policy advisers, sooner rather than later, like all previous U.S. governments, will become engaged in delicate world affairs.

However, the new government will soon be confronted with a major foreign policy dilemma that will never go away: the plight, and potential death of more than 25 million Africans living with HIV/AIDS. According to the United Nations agency that is coordinating the pandemic (UNAIDS), 25.3 million Africans live with the human immunodeficiency virus (HIV) that causes AIDS. Most of the infected are young men and women, 35 years or below, with small children, and at the prime productive stages of their lives. Every minute, 10 Africans contract the infection. Everyday in Africa, at least 5500 Africans die of AIDS. Since the beginning of the epidemic in the early 1980's, more than 17 million Africans have met their untimely deaths from the disease. Within the next 20 years, 41 million African children will become AIDS orphans, having lost one or both parents to the disease. In Botswana, 40 percent of its adult population are believed to be living with the HIV virus, and will likely die within a decade. Ten African nations have HIV/AIDS prevalence of 20 percent or more. To summarize, many African nations are under the vice grip of a ferocious disease that steals its young, sentences its very young to a life without parents, and burdens its elderly with the exhaustive task of simultaneously fending for themselves and their orphaned grandchildren.

An AIDS ravaged Africa cannot trade with any nation, practice effective democracy, enforce peacekeeping obligations, reform its economic systems or guarantee social justice. The World Bank and the United Nations projects that the reeling African economy will further decline by 25 percent within 15 years from AIDS. By 2015, many African countries will lose 30 years of their projected life expectancy to AIDS. As breadwinners die prematurely of AIDS, the struggle for scarce resources in Africa will intensify, and many nation states may disintegrate. Africa, as we know it, may cease to exist if sustained assistance is not forthcoming.

Africans should benefit from the Bush Administration's "compassionate" disposition. As an administration that touts compassion as a guiding principle, the plight of 25 million Africans living under a death sentence should elicit immediate and sustained response. For the next twelve months, as the global print and electronic media entities and energized civil society organizations focus on the plight of African AIDS victims, the Bush Administration will find it extremely difficult to ignore the precarious situation in Africa. The new administration will be called upon to demonstrate leadership in the following areas:

Resolving to maintain a strong political will on ending the epidemic. A clear signal will be the continued retention and operations of the White House Office on HIV/AIDS.

Resolving the current impasse over access to lifesaving drugs for African HIV/AIDS patients. The UNAIDS estimates that an African AIDS patient will require between $1,400 and $4,200 a year to access lifesaving antiretroviral drugs. Some generic manufacturers are pledging to provide these drugs at much reduced prices if they receive approval from the original pharmaceutical patent holders.

Funding prevention programs at community levels. The UNAIDS estimates that Africa needs $3 billion annually for effective preventive programs, yet only $300 million is spent.

Reducing the debt of African nations. African countries are saddled with massive foreign debt repayment schedules ($15 billion a year) that significantly reduce outlays for health, education, food, and basic infrastructure. Some countries spend more money on debt repayments than their combined expenditure on healthcare and education. The Bush Administration will have to push the G-8 for major debt relief for African governments.

Rebuilding the healthcare infrastructure. Africa's healthcare system is tottering towards collapse from a combination of mismanagement, political neglect, and the onslaught of AIDS. In some African countries, AIDS patients account for 60 percent of all hospitalizations. The UNAIDS estimates that one year of basic medical costs for a person with AIDS is equivalent to two to three times a country's average yearly GDP per capita. According to the World Bank, a serious national HIV/AIDS program will require 1.5-2.0 percent of that nation's GDP.

22

COMBATING HIV/AIDS IN AFRICA: AFRICA NEEDS FINANCIAL RELIEF, NOT COMMERCIAL LOANS

(July, 2000)

The Export-Import Bank of the United States (Ex-Im Bank), after months of searching for a role in the crystallizing global efforts to combat the HIV/AIDS pandemic in Africa, announced July 19, 2000 that it will provide $1 billion a year in five-year "term financing" to support the purchase of U.S. HIV/AIDS medication and related equipment by Sub-Saharan Africa nations. According to the Press Release for the event, Ex-Im Bank will "cooperate" with several pharmaceutical giants - including those companies that had previously announced various initiatives to assist African countries obtain medicines at cheaper prices - to ensure that HIV/AIDS patients will have access to lifesaving drugs. In addition, the Bank reported that representatives of unnamed African governments strongly support the proposed financing mechanism.

Slated to benefit from the Ex-Im Bank financing are the following countries: Benin, Botswana, Burkina Faso, Cameroon, Cape Verde, Côte d'Ivoire, Gabon, The Gambia, Ghana, Kenya, Lesotho, Mali, Mauritius, Mozambique, Namibia, Niger, Nigeria, Senegal, Seychelles, South Africa, Swaziland, Tanzania, Uganda, and Zimbabwe. According to the Ex-Im Bank, the proposed "pilot" program will add "flexibility," "minimize the cost," and "maximize the repayment terms" of the loan. In plain language, the Ex-Im Bank will enter into a commercial relationship with poor African countries that are facing the biggest threat to their corporate existence - the menace of the deadly HIV/AIDS that leaves death and destruction in its wake. The projected $1,000 to $2,000 annual price for the life saving drugs in Africa through the proposed financing, though a significant reduction from the present cost of these drugs is still way beyond the capacities of many national governments and peoples of Africa.

Despite the good intentions of Ex-Im Bank, since it is a credit agency and not a donor organization, I believe that any mechanism that will increase the aggregate financial burden of poor African countries will have very little effect on the epidemic. To explore this observation, it may be necessary to review the current state of development indicators for Africa.

The Current State of Africa

Africa represents 10 percent of the world population but accounts for 71 percent of all persons living with HIV/AID. The number of HIV/AIDS patients in Africa is at least 25 million; at least 13 million Africans have died of AIDS in Africa; Africans unduly suffer from the six big killer diseases: Malaria, HIV/AIDS, Tuberculosis, Measles, diarrhoeal diseases, and acute respiratory infections. The loss of man-hours is incalculable, and the preventable deaths from these conditions, tragic.

At least 290 million Africans, more than the entire U.S. population, survive on $1 a day, the cost of a no-name cup of coffee in the United States. A recent report from the World Bank suggests that many African countries are worse off today compared to 35 or 40 years ago when they won their independence; the national wealth of hardest-hit African countries, especially in Southern Africa, will be reduced by 15-20 percent because of HIV/AIDS.

The total combined income for the 48 countries in Africa is just above that of Belgium; the economies of many African countries are smaller than that of a typical small town of 60,000 persons in an industrialized country.

Some African countries have staggering debt, at 100 percent of national income. Nigeria is a prime example. The United Nations Development Program (UNDP) in its 1997 *Annual Report* concluded that African governments can save the lives of millions of children by 2000 if the international financial institutions can relieve the governments of debt obligations. Aid agencies have concluded that in the 40 poorest nations, 13 children die every 60 seconds because of national policies that divert financial resources from social welfare programs to debt repayments. Africa is the most indebted region in the world.

Eighty percent of Africans lack access to electricity, and 75 percent of rural Africans lack basic sanitation and access to clean drinking water. The information superhighway is yet to take root in Africa as the continent has the lowest rates of telephone usage, Internet connection, and other forms of telecommunications compared to any other region. In this era of globalization, telecommunications is a major tool for efficient commerce and international relationships.

Africa, clearly, is not in a financial position to enter into commercial agreements that will require strict repayment schedules and obligations while combating the complex direct and collateral consequences of HIV/AIDS. Without rehashing the well-known statistics about the epidemiology of HIV/AIDS in Africa, it is evident that Africa is in the throes of a major catastrophe. Virtually all the countries slated to receive funding from the Ex-Im Bank are either awaiting debt relief from the G-8 nations or campaigning for it. HIV/AIDS is a global emergency that deserves global, unrestricted response.

Suggested Remedial Action

African governments should shun any commercial agreement to purchase HIV/AIDS drugs. The international community - the public and private sector - should make these drugs available to needy nations in Africa. The international community should work out the financing mechanisms, and African governments will ensure that the drugs reach the intended individuals. The international community should help fund the annual $3 billion price tag for an effective HIV/AIDS prevention program in Africa.

African governments must develop and implement an effective HIV/AIDS strategy for their countries. The culture of denial must end. African governments should revamp their health care system. The primary, secondary, and tertiary health care systems should be reorganized, properly funded, and managed. The organized business sector in African countries should become strong allies in national efforts to control the epidemic. For example, the oil companies in Nigeria should become very active in the HIV/AIDS control efforts in the Niger Delta area.

I am a firm believer that a serious national government can mobilize its private sector during a period of emergency. African governments, as a matter of priority, should investigate all claims of palliative and/or clinical remedies for HIV/ADS by their medical practitioners and other citizens. No effort should be spared to develop effective remedies for the disease. The race to find a cure for HIV/AIDS should be of outmost concern to all Africans.

The HIV/AIDS problem in Africa is a humanitarian one. It deserves an uncomplicated humanitarian response with Africans and the international community working together. The U.S. Export-Import Bank, its counterpart export credit agencies and other multilateral institutions can devise creative ways for assisting African nations without saddling them with additional debts. If 25 million people in the United States or Britain face certain death from a disease, the responsible agencies will find a way to assist these individuals.

23

PRESIDENTIAL POLITICS AND THE DEAFENING SILENCE ON THE HIV/AIDS CRISIS IN AFRICA

(November, 2000)

The race for the White House is living up to the billing as one of the closest in American history. Vice President Al Gore and Governor George Bush alternate tiny leads in opinion polls. Pundits in the print and electronic media are having a field day discussing key policy issues that may influence the outcome of the election. The consensus is that foreign policy will be in the mind of voters as they head to the polls, especially with the televised images of the escalating Arab/Israel conflict. The pundits also believe that the rising energy costs, the change of guard in Yugoslavia and future relations with the West, relationships with Russia, and the control of North Korea's missile technology are important foreign policy issues.

However, both presidential candidates and the media appear to maintain a studied, deafening silence on what may become the most important foreign policy dilemma for the incoming president: the unfolding AIDS crisis in Africa. According to the United Nations agency that is coordinating efforts to tackle the pandemic (UNAIDS), nearly 25 million African children, youth, young men and women live with the human immunodeficiency virus (HIV) that causes the fatal disease known as the acquired immunodeficiency syndrome (AIDS). Every minute, 11 people worldwide contract the infection, 10 of them in Africa. More than one-tenth of the adult population aged 15-49 in 16 African countries lives with the HIV virus. Every day in Africa, 5,500 families will lose a loved one to AIDS. More than 12 million Africans have died of AIDS, and 10 million will die within the next ten years. A quarter of the entire population of Southern Africa will likely die of AIDS. By 2020, 41 million African children will become AIDS orphans, having lost one or both parents to the disease. Infected babies in Africa represent 95 percent of all maternal transmissions in the world. In a hospital in South Africa, the Baragwanath Hospital in Soweto, 40 percent of the 600 babies delivered every month are HIV positive.

Africa as we know it has the potential to become a wasteland as its best and brightest die at their prime, and leave their young children to harried relatives and extended family members. A recent documentary on HIV/AIDS in Africa by Rory Kennedy, the daughter of Robert Kennedy, showed a poor grandmother in Uganda taking care of 35 grandchildren after losing all but one of her nine children to AIDS. Because of the sheer magnitude of AIDS, the famed African extended family system is under strain. Yet, the unfolding tragedy in Africa is barely attracting attention in the presidential campaign. During the three presidential debates, neither the moderator nor the presidential candidates discussed the plight of nearly 25 million Africans living on death row. These infected Africans will die since they are unlikely to have access to life-saving drugs that has changed the face of AIDS in this country and other Western democracies. It is estimated that only 20,000 AIDS patients in Africa have access to life-saving drugs.

Africa often gets a passing reference in this presidential campaign with exhortations on how America will help fund peace keeping operations, enhance "conflict resolution", encourage macroeconomic reforms and trade liberalization, and institutionalize democratic ideas. However noble these ideas may be, the HIV/AIDS pandemic can upend them. To make this point clearer, I will briefly review the potential consequences of this terrible disease.

Conflicts in Africa

The root cause of all major conflicts in Africa is the constant struggle for scarce resources. Where these resources appear plentiful, such as large deposits of oil and diamonds, they are often in the hands of non-Africans and their tiny, corrupt, elite African collaborators. These struggles may be couched in ethnic, religious, social, or political terms. However, they remain essentially a primordial struggle for the control of these resources because of the winner-takes-all mentality of African leaders and their followers. The HIV/AIDS pandemic will exacerbate these struggles as millions of young men and women die and the tenuous social fabric of communities in Africa implodes from significant proportions of poor grandparents assuming responsibility for their orphaned grandchildren.

Macroeconomic Reforms and Trade Liberalization in Africa

This is already a casualty of the HIV/AIDS debacle. According to studies conducted by the World Bank and the United Nations, the African economy will decline by 25 percent within 15 years from the pandemic. During the same period, some African countries will lose 30 years of their peoples' projected life expectancy to AIDS. Rapid declines in life expectancy portend grave risks of social revolutions, ethnic schisms, and genocide. This is unfortunate because of the current fragile state of the Africa economy. Agriculture, the mainstay of rural economies in Africa, is already reeling from the unprecedented AIDS-related deaths of farmers, agricultural engineers, agronomists, and experienced farming helps.

The expected trade relationship between Africa and the U.S. depends on healthy, prosperous customers and exporters, an unlikely scenario with the AIDS pandemic. Hard-won gains in primary and secondary school enrollment are under threat as pupils are withdrawn from schools to care for dying parents or to become breadwinners for their families. School enrollment is also eroding from the high numbers of teachers that are infected or dying of AIDS. According to a recent report from the United Nations Children's Fund, an estimated 860,000 African schoolchildren lost their teachers to AIDS in 1999, and in the first 10 months of 1998, two-thirds of new teachers (1,300) in Zambia died of AIDS.

Democracy

The HIV/AIDS epidemic will end nascent African democracies for many reasons. First, the military of many African countries have high rates of HIV infection (30-50 percent), and are unlikely to tolerate lack of access to life saving drugs for their officer corps. The itch to forcibly take over power and ensure access to scarce national resources will be strong as popular military officers die of AIDS. Second, most countries with high rates of HIV/AIDS also have high rates of infant deaths, another major foe of democracy. High rates of infant deaths in any jurisdiction suggest huge disparities in socioeconomic and environmental conditions, a fertile ground for insurrection. Third, population-based democratic practices cannot take root in the presence of internecine struggle for power and control of resources, revolutions, and ethnic schisms. Finally, AIDS is wiping out the educated young men and women in Africa that are expected to be the harbingers of democracy.

The next U.S. president will face major domestic and foreign policy challenges. The candidates have done their best to sharpen the differences in their domestic agenda. Regarding foreign policy issues, both candidates appear united in saying that "national interests" will remain paramount in overseas engagements. It is unlikely that an American president will ignore the plight of 25 million Africans living under a death sentence. Ordinary Americans support sustained U.S. attention to the HIV/AIDS pandemic in Africa. According to the May/June Kaiser Family Foundation national survey of "American Views on the AIDS Crisis in Africa," more than six of every ten Americans (64 percent) support using federal funds to help solve the HIV/AIDS problem in Africa. It is a mystery why Gore and Bush have maintained a studied silence on the fate of nearly 25 million Africans on death row.

Both candidates should publicly state their positions on the following HIV/AIDS issues in Africa:

(1) Access to lifesaving drugs for HIV/AIDS patients: Less than 1 percent of infected Africans have access to these drugs, and no African country can afford the expensive treatment despite pledges of significant price reductions by pharmaceutical companies. UNAIDS estimates that it will cost between $1,400 and $4,200 a year

per patient to provide lifesaving drugs in Africa. America will have to lead the way for an international, Marshall Plan- type response.

(2) Funding for information, education, and communication (IEC) campaigns: The UNAIDS estimates that it will cost $3 billion annually for IEC and other prevention activities. Currently, only $300 million is spent.

(3) Reducing maternal transmission: African countries have had to make painful choices between allocating scarce resources for proven methods that reduce maternal transmission of HIV and expenditure on other health problems such as malaria, tuber-culosis, and sexually transmitted diseases. However, recent studies suggest that the drug Nevirapine, combined with no breastfeeding, can significantly reduce maternal transmission at a fraction of the cost of other expensive treatments. Ironically, after two decades of promoting breastfeeding, African governments are grappling with the tradeoff between the advantages of breastfeeding and the disadvantages of HIV infection.

(4) Funding for orphan children: Orphanage care is not only very expensive ($2,000 per child annually) but also culturally impracticable. The U.S. Agency for International Development (AID) estimates that it will cost $100 per year to keep a child in a kinship environment or within the extended family system.

(5) Revamping the healthcare infrastructure: Virtually every African country labors under failed or failing healthcare clinics, hospitals, and diagnostic centers. Most countries have lost their experienced medical and allied health staff to health institutions in the West and the Middle East. The financial burden of HIV/AIDS is high. According to UNAIDS, one year of basic medical costs for a person with AIDS is equivalent to two to three times a country's average yearly GDP per capita. The World Bank estimates that a serious national HIV/AIDS program will require 1.5-2.0 percent of that nation's GDP.

(6) Engaging the civil society: Most African countries run command-and-control economic and political programs with limi-ted participation of non-government organizations. The HIV/AIDS pandemic requires equal participation of the civil society and the government in the design, implementation, monitoring, and evaluation of HIV/AIDS programs. The U.S. and its allies will play a

crucial role in accelerating democratic reforms in Africa and encouraging African governments to collaborate with their civil society. Ironically, the HIV/AIDS onslaught may represent a window of opportunity for significant democratic reforms in Africa.

(7) Reducing Poverty: The HIV infection thrives in conditions of poverty. At least 290 million Africans, more than the entire population of America, live on under one dollar a day. Despite the grinding poverty, Africa spends $15 billion servicing its external debts to Western-based institutions. Some countries spend more money on debt repayments than their combined expenditure on healthcare and education.

Selected Bibliography

Chinua Akukwe (1999). "HIV/AIDS in African Children: A Major Calamity That Deserves Urgent Global Action." *Journal of HIV/AIDS Prevention and Education for Adolescents and Children*. Vol. 3, No. 3, pages 5-23.

Chinua Akukwe (2000). "Responding to the Pandemic of HIV/AIDS." Paper presented at the Foreign Affairs Brain trust, 30th Congressional Black Caucus Conference, September, Washington, DC.

Barton Cellman, "AIDS Is Declared Threat to Security. " *Washington Post* April 30, 2000, pages 1, 28, 29.

Barton Cellman. "Death Watch: The Global Response to AIDS in Africa. World Shunned Signs of the Coming Plague," *Washington Post* June 5, 2000; "Death Watch: South Africa's Response to AIDS," *Washington Post* July 6, 2000; "Death Watch: An African Community Response. Disease Far Outpaced the News," *Washington Post* July 7, 2000.

UNAIDS (2000). *Report on the Global HIV/AIDS Epidemic-June 2000*. Geneva. June. www.unaids.org

UNAIDS (2000). Press Release 2000: "AIDS Devastates Health Sector in Africa. African Ministers Meet to Intensify Efforts Against Epidemic." Geneva. May. www.unaids.org

USAID (2000). Children on the Brink. Washington, DC.

UNICEF (2000). *Annual Progress of Nations*. New York.

World Bank (2000). *Can Africa Claim the 21st Century?* Washington, DC.

World Bank (1998). *Intensifying Action Against HIV/AIDS in Africa: Responding to a Development Crisis*. Washington, DC.

National Summit on Africa (2000). *National Policy Plan of Action for U.S.-Africa Relations in the 21st Century*. Washington, DC.

Kaiser Family Foundation (2000). *American Views on AIDS Crisis in Africa*. Menlo Park, CA.

24

HIV/AIDS IN AFRICA: TIME TO STOP THE KILLING FIELDS

With Melvin Foote
(April, 2001)

Introduction

According to the UN Agency for HIV/AIDS (UNAIDS), 25.3 million Africans live with the virus or are dying of AIDS. Barring a miracle or a major change in international attention to the scourge, these Africans will die within the next decade. Despite the horrors of the pandemic, the international responses have been limited and only recently have most African governments begun to publicly address the problem. African governments are hobbled by poverty, cultural taboos about sex, and misperceptions about the cause and seriousness of AIDS. They also fear disruption of precious tourism and investment dollars from the West and have failed to warn their citizens about the dangers of AIDS. Western nations, including the U.S., have largely ignored the dangers and international repercussions of widespread infection in Africa. The United States in 2000 spent only $300 million for basic AIDS care and prevention programs in Africa—far short of the $3 billion regarded as necessary to slow down the pandemic.

The HIV/AIDS crisis in Africa is of the gravest magnitude. Every day, 6,700 families lose a loved one to the disease; the construction and sale of coffins is one of the fastest growing occupations in southern Africa. Sixteen African countries have one-tenth or more of their population infected with HIV, and Africa is home to 95 percent of all mother-to-child transmissions of HIV. In these countries, almost 80 percent of all deaths of young adults aged 25-45 will be directly linked to AIDS.

In six countries of southern Africa, by the year 2005, AIDS will claim the lives of between 8 percent and 25 percent of today's active physicians. Women are affected more by this dreaded disease; in Africa, 12 women have HIV/AIDS for every 10 men. African women account for 85 percent of all global female infections. In southern Africa, one in four women aged 15-49 live with HIV/AIDS. In some countries, between 10 percent and 20 percent of teenage girls are already infected. Infected girls are more likely than boys to drop out of school, reversing decades of slow but steady progress in female education. The much-vaunted African extended family system is faltering, as the number of orphans living without the care of extended families rises. By the year 2010, the projected number of orphans may exceed 40 million in Africa.

Africa's hard-won health and education gains in the 1960s and 1970s were undermined by debt and by externally dictated structural adjustment policies in the 1980s and 1990s. Today, however, social services and economies are imploding from the deadly consequences of AIDS. In the coming decades, the continent will record significantly sharper declines in life expectancy rates and shrinkage of national economies from the effects of the epidemic.

Africans living with HIV/AIDS have limited or no access to lifesaving anti-retroviral medicines that have changed the course and management of AIDS in Western countries. Less than one-tenth of one percent of Africans living with AIDS have access to AIDS drugs. The World Bank estimates that half of all Africans live on $0.65 cents per day. The economic resources of African governments are equally meager, and they are burdened by $20 billion in annual foreign debt payments. With the rudimentary healthcare infrastructure of African countries, the strain of long-term hospitalization of AIDS patients is taking a heavy toll.

Economic underdevelopment and Africa's impoverished conditions have created a wide-open gateway for HIV infection, tuberculosis (TB), and sexually transmitted diseases (STDs). According to the World Health Organization, an estimated 30-50 percent of all TB patients in Africa are also infected with HIV/AIDS.

Africa has the highest rates of STDs in the world. STDs facilitate the spread of HIV infection, especially among women.

Political instability and violent conflicts keep many African governments from focusing on the

AIDS crisis. Twenty of the continent's 53 countries are involved in intrastate or interstate conflicts, which lead to having the world's largest regional concentration of refugees. Another important factor in the deepening crisis is the high rate of AIDS within Africa's armed forces—15-20 percent of the members of the military in some countries have AIDS. Mobility of the African male populations through military operations, migrant labor such as mine workers, and shifts from rural to urban centers—exacerbates the spread of HIV/AIDS. As the HIV/AIDS pandemic continues, political and social instability will likely intensify as AIDS gobbles up scarce human and economic resources.

Problems with Current U.S. Policy

Key Problems

The U.S. has not provided global leadership on access to AIDS drugs for Africa and has not supported Africa's demand to purchase or produce generic drugs. The U.S. 2001 budget for fighting AIDS in Africa is about $460 million, but much more is needed. The U.S. has yet to assert its influence at the World Bank and the IMF to put more resources in Africa and to cancel external debts.

Whether someone lives or dies of AIDS depends largely on where she or he lives. Despite the availability of drugs to treat AIDS, millions of Africans will die because they do not have access to AIDS drugs. In the U.S. and other Western nations, such drugs have helped AIDS to become a disease that can be managed and for which effective care is available.

Confronting the AIDS emergency, African governments are demanding that pharmaceutical companies directly provide AIDS drugs at deep discounts, or at the very least not oppose compulsory licensing and parallel import arrangements. Compulsory licensing is an international trade mechanism by which countries can instruct a patent holder to license the right to use this patent to any national company or government agency. Parallel importing describes a practice whereby a country imports goods for resale without authorization from the original seller. This struggle became heated with the court battle between the government of South Africa and 39 drug companies. The companies contended that a new law would allow the South African government to ignore international patent law.

Under mounting international pressure, the pharmaceutical industry dropped its suit, and has promised to facilitate the flow of low-priced AIDS-treatment pharmaceuticals. But this issue will not go away, because even lower priced drugs will still be out of reach for most Africans, and the pharmaceutical industry remains committed to strong international patent protection and to staving off the production of generic medicines for the treatment of AIDS and other illnesses.

The U.S. and its Western allies have failed to provide significant funds to fight AIDS in Africa. In 2001, the wealthiest nation on earth is spending only 460 million dollars to fight the biggest medical and humanitarian emergency of our time. The United Nations estimates that at least $10 billion will be needed to fight AIDS in Africa. A group of Harvard researchers, economists, and scientists recommended that, at a bare minimum, the U.S. should spend $1.5 billion a year to fight AIDS in Africa.

Fortunately, U.S. policymakers are responding to such public pressure with increased allocations. The U.S. Senate, for example, recently approved a $700 million increase in proposed spending over the next two years to fight AIDS in poor countries. However, much more needs to be done.

In another major issue confronting Africa, U.S. policymakers have not squared up to their responsibility. Africa owes foreign banks and governments about $350 billion. These debts are controversial and a major hindrance to an adequate African response to AIDS. Every year, Africa spends roughly $20 billion on debt repayment—more than the combined continental outlay for healthcare and education. At least 23 African countries spend more money on debt repayment than they spend for healthcare. The International Monetary Fund (IMF) and the World Bank have yet to effect significant debt cancellation for African nations despite widespread pressure from international citizen movements and from the G8, the forum of the world's wealthiest nations. The U.S., which is the largest shareholder in these two international financial institutions, has yet to demand debt cancellation for Africa.

The policy problems that contribute to the AIDS crisis in Africa extend beyond Washington and other international donors. Until recently, African leaders have largely ignored the pandemic. Even today, very few African nations match their AIDS rhetoric with commensurate budget allocations. Uganda and Senegal are prominent exceptions.

Senegal, through a combination of political will, prudent budget allocations, and massive mobilization has kept its rate of infection to less than one percent. Ugandan President Yoweri Museveni, recognizing the gravity of the AIDS pandemic, mobilized his people to modify risky behavior and to come forward for testing and counseling. The rate of AIDS in Uganda is down to about 8 percent, from a high of 16 percent in the early 1990s. Despite the laudable efforts of Uganda and Senegal, corruption and the squandering of scarce national resources continue. Government spending on wars, white elephant projects, and persecution of political and economic opponents is still rife across the continent.

Toward a New Foreign Policy:

Key Recommendations

The U.S. should lead other rich nations in supplying essential medicines to Africans living with AIDS, and devote significantly more resources to fighting AIDS in Africa;

The U.S. should lead the fight for debt relief for African nations and ensure that the savings go into AIDS relief and other healthcare programs;

The U.S. and other rich nations should work with African governments to create an environment conducive to AIDS relief on the continent.

The immediate goal of a reinvigorated U.S. policy should be the dismantling of all legal and logistic obstacles to the provision of affordable drugs to all Africans living with AIDS. The developed nations, led by the U.S., should rise in unison and make a simple pledge: No African Man, Woman, Child, or Infant Should Be Denied Access to Lifesaving AIDS Drugs, by December 2002.

As the leading global democracy, the U.S. should democratize access to essential AIDS medicines for poor nations. We commend the Bush administration for maintaining President Clinton's executive order on flexible access to AIDS drugs for poor nations. However, the U.S. needs to do more. The U.S. should ensure that the World Trade Organization (WTO) implements a flexible interpretation of the Trade-Related Intellectual Property Rights Agreement (TRIPS), thereby allowing poor nations facing the AIDS emergency to provide cheap AIDS drugs to their citizens. The U.S. and its allies should also ensure that all WTO rulings reflect a sound public health framework to ensure that the goal of unencumbered trade does not create adverse health consequences in poor nations.

The U.S. government should work more closely with the pharmaceutical companies to ensure that all obstacles to speedy and effective delivery of AIDS medicines to poor nations are eliminated. These obstacles include: (1) the concerns of pharmaceutical companies about possible parallel imports of cheap AIDS drugs into the lucrative Western markets by poor nations; (2) the concerns of citizen advocates and AIDS activists that access to AIDS drugs should not come under the purview of market forces and restrictive patent laws; and, (3) the concerns of African governments that they should have the exclusive prerogative to determine national emergencies and possible remedial actions. Washington should also work to persuade U.S. multinational companies doing business in Africa to provide AIDS prevention and treatment programs for their workers and family members.

The U.S. should devote more resources to fighting AIDS in Africa. America has always responded to major humanitarian needs, whether in Europe, Asia, or Latin America. It is time to spend readily available resources to stop AIDS in Africa. Harvard researchers estimated that a scaled-up U.S. response of $1.5 billion would cost about $5 a year per American. Doubling such a commitment would cost each American about $10 a year—a commitment well worth making, considering the magnitude of the crisis and its long-term implications for global peace and development.

It is not likely that other rich nations will spend significantly more money on AIDS without a serious commitment from the United States. The Constituency for Africa (CFA), under the leadership of former Congressman Ron Dellums, proposed a HIV/AIDS Marshall Plan for Africa with significant public- and private-sector funds to fight the disease. As a result, Congress, in August 2000, passed Public Law 106-264, the Global AIDS and Tuberculosis Relief Act of 2000, sponsored by Jim Leach, R-Iowa and Barbara Lee, D-California that earmarked 150 million dollars for each of the fiscal years 2001 and 2002, for a Trust Fund. The Trust Fund will be used to leverage funds from multilateral development banks like the World Bank and to encourage similar commitments from other Western donors. The Trust Fund will also fund the implementation of specific HIV/AIDS programs in Africa. President Clinton signed the bill into law, as a modest start to what promises to be a long journey.

The U.S. should use its significant leverage in the G8, the IMF, and the World Bank to provide debt relief for African nations. The U.S. has the excellent opportunity at the G8 summit, in July 2001, to persuade its allies to forgive the debt of African nations, on the condition that African governments plow back such savings into verifiable investments in AIDS prevention and treatment programs and other healthcare services. The U.S. government is not the major holder of African debt—it is owed about $360 million out of the estimated $350 billion in controversial debts—but the U.S. has the moral, economic, and political leverage to advance a genuine debt relief agenda among its allies. Washington should also work with African leaders and their peoples to ensure a concerted and consistent focus on the AIDS epidemic. Without dictating their actions, the U.S. should work with African governments to ensure movement in the following areas: (1) allocation of more money by African nations to fight AIDS; (2) sustained political reforms to encourage pluralistic political and multi-sector campaigns against AIDS; (3) end corrupt practices that siphon foreign aid and investments; and, (4) encourage the emergence of more civil society involvement in politics and non-government programs at community levels.

The international community led by the U.S. should not turn its back on 25 million Africans living under a death sentence. The international cooperation that has fought against oppression and tyranny since World War II should not permit the AIDS killing fields to continue in Africa. A strong case can be made that the AIDS pandemic in Africa represents a direct threat to U.S. national interests and national security because of associated political instability, economic downturn, and the intercontinental spread of infectious diseases. In the end, however, U.S. citizens and U.S. policymakers face a moral imperative and should ask: Have we done all we can to save 25 million fellow human beings from an avoidable death?

Selected Bibliography

Chinua Akukwe, "AIDS and Men: Taking Risks or Taking Responsibility?" *Journal of the Royal Society for the Promotion of Health*, March 2000, 120 (1).

Chinua Akukwe, "Africa's HIV/AIDS Dilemma," *The Washington Times*, November 26, 2000.

Chinua Akukwe, "HIV/AIDS in African Children: A Major Calamity that Deserves Urgent Global Action," *Journal of HIV/AIDS Prevention and Education for Adolescents and Children*, 1999, 3 (3).

Chinua Akukwe, "The Need for an Urban HIV/AIDS Policy in the United States," *Journal of Health and Social Policy*, 2001, 12 (3).

Gro Harlem Brundtland, "Affordable AIDS Drugs are Within Reach," *The International Herald Tribune*, February 14, 2001. Dr Brundtland is the former Director General of the World Health Organization (WHO).

Melvin Foote and Chinua Akukwe, "Clinton's Visit to Nigeria: HIV/AIDS Should be at the Top of the Agenda," *The Constituency for Africa Policy Brief*, August 2000, Washington, DC.

Melvin Foote and Chinua Akukwe, "The Gains of the 13th International AIDS Conference in Durban, South Africa," *Africa Economic Analysis*, August 2000. Available at http://www.afbis.com

FPIF Editors, "Citizens-Based Global Affairs Agenda: Democratizing Access to Essential Medicines," *Foreign Policy in Focus*, March 2001. Available at http://www.fpif.org/cgaa/pharma.html.

Uwe Friesecke, "Globalization Left a Suffering Africa," Paper presented at the January 2001 Conference on "Peace through Development along the Nile Valley," Khartoum, Sudan, and reported in http://www.members.tripod.com, accessed March 2001.

General Accounting Office, "Global Health: U.S. Agency for International Development Fights AIDS in Africa, but Better Data Needed to Measure Impact," GAO-01-449, Washington, DC, 2001.

Jeffrey Sachs, "A Global Fund for the Fight Against AIDS," *The Washington Post*, Saturday, April 7, 2001.

UNAIDS and World Health Organization, *AIDS Epidemic Update: December 2000*, Geneva, Switzerland, 2000.

United Nations, Special Session of the General Assembly on HIV/AIDS, *Report of the Secretary General*, UN General Assembly, New York, February 16, 2001.

Robert Weissman, "AIDS and Developing Countries: Democratizing Access to Essential Medicines," *Foreign Policy in Focus*, Volume 4, Number 23, August 1999. Available at http://www.fpif.org/briefs/vol4/v4n23aids.html.

Robert Weissman, "AIDS and Developing Countries: Facilitating Access to Essential Medicines," *Foreign Policy in Focus*, Volume 6, Number 6, February 2001. Available at http://www.fpif.org/briefs/vol6/v6n06aids.html.

World Bank, *Can Africa Claim the 21st Century?* Washington, DC, 2000.

25

HIV/AIDS IN AFRICA: AFRICAN-
AFRICAN AMERICAN COOPERATION*

(September, 2002)

I wish to thank the Secretary of State, General Colin Powell for his continued support for the Secretary's Open Forum in the State Department as an avenue for exchange of ideas on crucial issues. As a member of the Board of Directors of the Constituency for Africa (CFA), Washington, DC, I am aware of Colin Powell's personal and professional commitment to HIV/AIDS remedial efforts in Africa. In addition, the Secretary of State is strongly committed to sustained cooperation and partnership between the peoples of the great continent of Africa and its brothers and sisters in the Diaspora, of which he is a prominent member. I wish to thank Allan Lang, the Chairman of the Secretary's Open Forum for making this event possible.

The HIV/AIDS crisis in Africa is shaping up to be a major defining issue of our time. With 21.5 million Africans already dead of AIDS and 28.5 million living with HIV/AIDS in Africa and almost certain to pass on within the next few years without active intervention, the international community is faced with a crisis of unimaginable proportions. As the current 11 million AIDS orphans in Africa swell to more than 20 million by the end of the decade in Africa, the future of the continent is at stake. HIV/AIDS can create a society of sick people around the world, and especially in Africa, who are unable to work, trade, teach, minister to the sick, maintain law and order, manage diplomatic relations, improve intellectual pursuits or propel their children to greater heights in life.

The HIV/AIDS crisis in Africa and the consequent international response will loom large as the present leaders of the world, including United States, come under the brutal gaze of history. Our children and their children will ask critical questions regarding the response of our leaders to the death of millions of people from a disease that is not only preventable but also clinically manageable with currently available medicines and support services. The next generation will likely ask questions regarding the response of African leaders to the greatest development crisis under their watch. They will also ask questions regarding the response of the richest nations on earth, including the United States. They are also likely to ask questions on the response of the richest and the most powerful nation on Earth, the United States of America.

The HIV/AIDS crisis will also raise questions on what kind of society will allow a situation whereby 28.5 million people in Africa will die when resources are readily available for remedial measures. The crisis will raise questions on what kind of society will allow $7-10 billion a year to stand between a sustained and effective response to the HIV/AIDS crisis. These questions are already being raised, even from the highest policy makers. Last week, I had the honor of serving as the moderator of the late Honorable Ron Brown Lecture Series on HIV/AIDS in Africa, organized during the Congressional Black Caucus week in Washington, DC, with Dr Peter Piot, the executive director of UNAIDS as the keynote speaker. Dr Peter Piot made it very clear that the response to the HIV/AIDS crisis in Africa, both within Africa and from the international community, will be a major test of our moral, financial, intellectual, and policy values.

In my view, critical to the global response to the HIV/AIDS in Africa are two important constituencies: Africans and African-Americans. Both Africans and African Americans are at the receiving end of the epidemic, with African American women accounting for the fastest rising incidence of HIV infection in the United States. The AIDS quadrangle of poverty, tuberculosis, sexually transmitted diseases and HIV infection is endemic in the African-American community.

The African-American community played a strong role in mobilizing government's financial and technical resources for AIDS remedial effort in the urban centers of America with the strong support and participation of the Congressional Black Caucus. They also played a prominent role in pushing the Clinton and Bush administrations to mobilize resources for HIV/AIDS activities in Africa. The Constituency for Africa (CFA), the organization I serve as a board member, with the prompting of its chairman, Honorable Ron Dellums, made the HIV/AIDS crisis in Africa the central issue of its advocacy efforts in the United States through the AIDS Marshall Plan for Africa. It is also not a coincidence that Kofi Annan, the Secretary-General of the United Nations, a native of Ghana, practically dragged the international community kicking and screaming into developing a political response to the pandemic, culminating in the establishment of a global fund to tackle HIV/AIDS, Malaria and Tuberculosis in Africa and other parts of the world.

African-African American cooperation is crucial in mobilizing resources in Africa and energizing a strong coalition for AIDS relief in the West, especially in the United States. Since AIDS remedial efforts in Africa remain considerably slowed down by lack of resources, the envisaged African-African American cooperation must extend beyond slogans and empty rhetoric. The African-African American cooperation must have specific goals, specific timelines, and specific strategies as the clock ticks on the millions of Africans awaiting untimely death from AIDS. In 2001, I co-authored an article with Melvin Foote, the president of CFA on the need for an African-American agenda in the fight against HIV/AIDS in Africa. I will incorporate some of our conclusions in articulating what I consider to be goals for an African-African American agenda in the global fight against HIV/AIDS.

Ten Goals for an African-African-American Agenda

(1) Every African living with HIV/AIDS should have access to lifesaving antiretroviral therapy on or before December 2003.

(2) Every African pregnant woman should have access to life saving medicines that can reduce or eliminate mother-to-child transmission of HIV on or before March 2003.

(3) Every African AIDS orphan should be in school and receive appropriate medical care on or before December 2003.

(4) Every African nation must meet its commitment to devote 15 percent or more of their national budgets to health issues, including HIV/AIDS remedial efforts on or before December 2003.

(5) Every African nation should have enough resources to mount a credible information, education and communication campaign against HIV transmission on or before June 2003.

(6) The United States should contribute at least 50 percent or $5 billion needed every year in the global fight against HIV/AIDS, TB and malaria on or before December 2003.

(7) Every African country with 5 percent or more of its population living with HIV/AIDS should have its debts cancelled and the savings channeled to verifiable expenditures on health and social programs on or before June 2003.

(8) Every African country must demonstrate its commitment to population-based democracy, transparency in the rule of law, and the promotion of private enterprise in order to reduce concerns about governance in Africa and AIDS remedial efforts on or before June 2003.

(9) The New Partnership for Africa's Development (NEPAD) should have an action plan on HIV/AIDS on or before June 2003.

(10) On or before January 2004, a mechanism should be created whereby African professionals living in the West and African-American professionals can provide one or more years of volunteer or paid work in coordinated AIDS remedial efforts in Africa.

Each proposed goal for an African-African American agenda will address crucial issues in the fight against HIV/AIDS in Africa. Each goal can be translated into objectives and action steps that can mobilize human, material and technical resources. Each goal is also amenable to public and private partnerships, including civil society collaboration. As the clock ticks for the millions of Africans living on the AIDS death row, time is of the essence.

Remarks at the US Secretary of State Open Forum on African-African American Cooperation in the Global Fight Against HIV/AIDS, September 17, 2002, Washington, DC

26

HIV/AIDS IN AFRICA: IMPLICATIONS OF PRESIDENT BUSH'S EMERGENCY PLAN FOR AIDS RELIEF

With Melvin Foote
(February, 2003)

President Bush in his 2003 "State of the Union" address to US Congress announced the Emergency Plan for AIDS Relief initiative that will "commit 15 billion dollars over the next five years, including nearly ten billion dollars in new money, to turn the tide against AIDS in the most afflicted nations of Africa and the Caribbean." According to a White House Fact Sheet, the initiative will fund antiretroviral therapy for at least 2 million people, and help prevent 7 million new infections within the next five years in the following countries: Botswana, Ivory Coast, Ethiopia, Guyana, Haiti, Kenya, Mozambique, Namibia, Rwanda, Nigeria, South Africa, Tanzania, Uganda and Zambia.

Today, nearly 30 million people live with HIV/AIDS in Africa. More than 3 million Africans will likely become infected this year and more than two million are likely to die. For Africa, the President's pronouncement has multiple implications in the evolving battle against HIV/AIDS in the continent.

More money will likely be available to fight HIV/AIDS. If Congress approves and funds the Emergency Plan for AIDS Relief, it is likely that Europe will raise its contributions to AIDS remedial efforts in Africa to match or exceed U.S. contribution. Consequently, an outlay of $2 billion in U.S. backed AIDS relief can easily translate into Europe's commitment of $2 billion or more. UNAIDS estimates that Africa will require at least US$3 billion for AIDS care/support and another US$1.5 billion for prevention.

Boost in AIDS funding may not materialize in 2003. The Emergency Plan for AIDS Relief is expected to take off in 2004. Consequently, there may be no major increases in US financial support for 2003. Meanwhile, the AIDS epidemic and its destructive effects in Africa do not respect funding plans or orderly appropriation process.

Where will "old" money come from? As at the time of writing this article, we are unaware of the source of $5 billion in "old" money out of the projected $15 billion for the new initiative. We hope the "old" money will not lead to the sunset of current international HIV/AIDS programs. We also hope that the Millennium Challenge Account, whereby the U.S. is pledging to spend $5 billion dollars in development aid to the poorest countries, is not in jeopardy.

The future of the Global Fund for AIDS, TB and Malaria is up in the air. The new initiative will set aside $200 million a year for five years ($1 billion) for the Fund. Richard Feachem, the executive director of the Fund, recently stated at the January 2003 World Economic Forum meeting that his organization needs about US$ 6 billion by 2004 to meet anticipated commitments. The election of Tommy Thompson, US Secretary of Health and Human Services, as the new Chair of the Fund does not basically change the fact that the organization faces an imminent financial crunch.

Imminent end to the battle on access to cheap drugs. This may represent one of the most significant ramifications of the new initiative. By an unambiguous commitment to provide low cost anti-retroviral treatment to 2 million individuals, President Bush, in principle, wittingly or unwittingly, ended the dichotomy between access to generic and non-generic HIV/AIDS drugs. The combination of U.S. and Europe money for antiretroviral drugs will likely reduce the cost of these drugs to such a level that the quality of supplied drugs will supercede concerns about unit cost. We do not foresee a situation whereby research pharmaceutical companies or their lobby will stop a global effort led by the United States to provide the most cost-effective medical treatment to millions of individuals living with HIV/AIDS.

Prevention programs will be kick-started. Information, education and communication campaigns against HIV/AIDS in

Africa will receive a significant boost from the new initiative for two main reasons. First, improved and sustained access to life-saving medicines will shatter the current myth that AIDS is a definitive death sentence in Africa. Second, individuals who feel they are at risk will likely come forward for testing and counseling once they receive assurances that medical care is available.

Africa must deliver. If the U.S. and Europe come through with massive financial outlays for AIDS remedial efforts, African leaders and their citizens must do everything humanly possible to facilitate quality care and preventive programs in the continent. Africa will have to deliver on logistics of care, governance issues, community mobilization, monitoring and evaluation. To succeed in the fight against AIDS, Africa and its external friends must become indispensable partners, with each partner holding up its own end of the bargain. It is also crucial for Africa to mobilize its own resources (financial, technical, and cultural) to complement international remedial efforts.

African professionals in the West should take the initiative. Closely tied to more resources for AIDS remedial efforts in Africa and African governments getting their act together is the need for thousands of talented African professionals living and working in the West to answer the call for duty in the continent. A successful campaign against HIV/AIDS in Africa will require deployment of significant expertise in healthcare, development, politics, human rights and gender equity issues. We believe that African professionals living in the West will be crucial to any massive, global campaign to stop AIDS in Africa.

Civil society in the West may need to shift tactics. Although the new initiative is far short of the $10 billion a year needed to effectively tackle HIV/AIDS around the world, President Bush's dramatic announcement suggests that Western leaders are on the threshold of addressing the greatest development tragedy of our time. The passive/aggressive response of civil society to the new initiative suggests that it may be time to begin a strategic adjustment of priorities. First, civil society should have a contingency plan for the next steps if their financial or program targets are met. Second, civil society may need to put more emphasis on strengthening the capacity of their counterparts in

Africa to provide effective monitoring and evaluation of funded programs in the continent. Third, civil society may now set their targets on comprehensive reforms of delivery mechanisms such as multilateral agencies, to remove the last vestige of refuge for Western politicians and policy makers who cite implementation weaknesses of these agencies in their refusal to commit more resources for development emergencies.

Politics may creep into AIDS remedial efforts in Africa. The list of African countries slated to benefit from the Emergency Plan for AIDS Relief is commendable. However, we are struck by the absence of other heavily affected countries such as Zimbabwe (33.7 percent adult prevalence according to UNAIDS), Swaziland (33.4 percent), Lesotho (31 percent) and Malawi (15 percent). We hope that emergency AIDS remedial efforts will continue to be based on the epidemiology of the disease rather than international politics.

What happens to countries with current low rates of infection? The new initiative is focusing on heavily infected countries. However, the ultimate goal of remedial efforts is to prevent new infections or ensure that those already infected do not transmit the virus to other people. We hope that African countries with low rates of infection, such as most countries in North Africa, Senegal and Mauritius (2 percent or less) and others, will not be forgotten in international remedial efforts. Corporations will now be in the spotlight. A major plank of the initiative is "public/private" partnerships. Multinational corporations that do business in Africa are now in the spotlight regarding HIV/AIDS programs for their staff and families that live in their operational areas. International oil companies, mining/extraction companies, service organizations, and agricultural conglomerates will have to do more on HIV/AIDS in Africa. We commend the current efforts of the giant mining conglomerates in South Africa and Botswana to provide HIV/AIDS care and support services for their workers. However, as reluctant Western governments commit more money for AIDS remedial efforts in Africa, corporations will be under increasing scrutiny.

Foundations/philanthropic organizations will have to come through. As HIV/AIDS remedial efforts gathers momentum in Africa, foundations with deep pockets will have to come through to complement public and private sector activities. Foundations have major roles to play in funding comprehensive prevention programs; enhancing the capacity of communities struggling to take care of their infected sons and daughters; providing care and support for AIDS orphans; training community-based health workers; and supporting independent African-based research efforts on HIV/AIDS.

Can the U.S. end the link between poverty and HIV/AIDS? The Emergency Plan for AIDS Relief does not have any anti-poverty plank to the best of our knowledge. However, the linkage between abject poverty and transmission of HIV is well known. According to Africa Action of Washington, DC, African countries pay more than US$15 billion a year to international creditors every year. These debt payments sabotage genuine efforts to checkmate HIV/AIDS in heavily infected countries. We believe that debt relief for Africa tied to verifiable investments in HIV/AIDS programs will reenergize remedial efforts in the continent. We hope that President Bush will once again confound his critics by making another dramatic proposal on ending the draconian debts of African nations as part of the fight against HIV/AIDS.

Conclusion

President Bush's Emergency Plan for AIDS Relief is a step in the right direction. However, as with all bold pronouncements, the devil is in the details. Advocacy organizations, private entities, governments around the world and individuals living with or affected by HIV/AIDS will be watching with keen interest the action of Congress in the next few months. As the appropriation process takes its course, it is important to note that nearly 10, 000 Africans contract HIV every day, and almost 7,000 die of AIDS. For the millions clinging on to life, including 4 million that will benefit from immediate antiretroviral therapy, with every day we delay our assistance, it may be too little, too late for them and their families.

Selected Bibliography

Chinua Akukwe (2001). "HIV/AIDS in Africa: Unavoidable Foreign Policy Priority for Bush Administration." February 8, 2001. Available at http://allafrica.com/stories/printable/200102090287.html

President George W. Bush (2003). *State of the Union Address to Congress.* January 28, 2003. Available at http://whitehouse.gov/news/releases/2003/20030128-19html

White House (2003). *Countries that will Benefit from the U.S. Emergency Plan for AIDS Relief.* January 28. Available at http://allafrica.com/stories/printable/200301290193.html

Africa Action (2003). *Africa Policy for a New Era: Ending Segregation in U.S. Foreign Relations.* January 23, 2003. Executive Summary. Available at http://allafrica.com/stories/200301230864.html

World Economic Forum (2003). *Global Fund Calls for US$6 Billion More to Fight AIDS. January 28.* Available at http://allafrica.com/stories/printable/200301280813.html

UNAIDS (2002). *Report on the Global HIV/AIDS Epidemic.* 2002. Geneva: Author.

PART VI:

RETHINKING HIV/AIDS

STRATEGIES

27

THE NEED FOR AN INTERNATIONAL HIV/AIDS VOLUNTEER SERVICES CORPS FOR AFRICA

With Sidi Jammeh and George Haley
(January, 2005)

Africa is facing a formidable foe in HIV/AIDS. According to the latest report by the United Nations agency coordinating the global fight against the pandemic (UNAIDS), although Africa represents only 10 percent of the global population, it accounts for nearly 64 percent of HIV/AIDS worldwide - 25.4 million infected individuals, and counting. Africa is home to almost 76 percent of women living with HIV/AIDS worldwide. The southern region of Africa, which represents only 2 percent of the global population, is home to nearly 30 percent of the total number of persons living with HIV/AIDS worldwide. UNAIDS estimates that 2.3 million adults and children in Africa died of AIDS in 2004. Unlike the situation in North America, Europe, South America, and some countries in the Caribbean, where most people who need antiretroviral therapy receive the drugs, nine of every ten infected individuals in Africa that could benefit from these lifesaving drugs cannot access them.

Although remarkable successes have been recorded in the last few years in marshalling resources to fight the epidemic in Africa, a missing link has been the lack of a trained health and development workforce to successfully scale-up a multi-sectoral response in the continent. As we see it, there is a need for an international volunteer HIV/AIDS service corps that will tackle health and logistics challenges that impede a timely and effective response against HIV/AIDS in Africa. Our proposal does not envisage another global bureaucracy but will match skill sets with identified needs in various parts of Africa, and complement available services in at-risk areas in Africa.

Why an AIDS Volunteer Service Corps?

There are multiple reasons for a volunteer AIDS service corps in Africa. First, HIV/AIDS, although a health condition, has almost single-handedly reversed past development gains in Africa. According to UNAIDS, life expectancy in Africa today is 49 years instead of 62 years without HIV/AIDS. Nine countries in Africa currently have life expectancy rates of less than 40 years.

Second, 95 percent of UNAIDS offices in Africa, in a 2004 review, identified lack of health personnel as a major hindrance in the fight against AIDS. UNAIDS estimates that between 19 percent and 53 percent of all deaths among government health employees in Africa are directly attributable to AIDS. This situation is compounded by some of the lowest physician-to-population ratios in the world. According to the World Bank, there is one physician to every 35,000 persons in Ethiopia, with near similar ratios in many African nations. Health workers are laboring to cope with an unprecedented surge in the number of AIDS patients. In some hospitals in Africa, AIDS patients occupy more than 60 percent of all available beds. Furthermore, thousands of health workers have left Africa for more lucrative careers in the West. Although South Africa has the largest number of individuals living with HIV/AIDS, at least 5,000 doctors left South Africa in recent years, according to UNAIDS.

Third, the non-health workforce in Africa is also reeling from the effects of HIV/AIDS. The International Labor Organization, in a recent report, indicated that HIV/AIDS by 2000 accounted for nearly 12 percent of total labor losses in Zimbabwe and more than 10 percent in Zambia. Agriculture, the mainstay of Africa's economy (24 percent of the continent's GDP and 40 percent of its foreign exchange earnings) is under strain from HIV/AIDS. By 2020, AIDS may kill one fifth of all agricultural workers in Africa. AIDS is causing a shortage of teachers in Zambia and Zimbabwe. Businesses in the southern region of Africa sometimes hire two or more persons for the same job because of justified fears of losing a highly trained worker to AIDS.

Fourth, the healthcare infrastructure in Africa is reeling from years of inadequate funding and mismanagement. Community-based clinics need to be revamped, hospitals re-equipped, and training programs jumpstarted.

Fifth, funding constraints remain a major obstacle in AIDS remedial efforts in Africa. According to UNAIDS estimates, the total expenditure on AIDS worldwide in 2004 was about US$6.1 billion. By 2007, at least US$20 billion a year will be needed for an effective fight against the pandemic. Nearly 43 percent of the US$20 billion will be needed in Africa. A recent World Bank guide on widening access to lifesaving HIV/AIDS medicines in developing countries concluded that it would require considerable resources to close the gap between the need to treat millions of people living with HIV/AIDS and the low national healthcare budget of poor countries around the world.

Sixth, prevention programs, despite more than two decades of effort, have not been very effective. Prevention programs encompass information, education, and communication campaigns against selected health conditions, targeted at specific audiences and populations at risk. A recent survey by UNICEF indicates that up to 50 percent of young women in some countries with a high rate of HIV transmission are unaware of basic facts about the disease. Another survey of 73 low and middle income countries (most of them in Africa), which account for more than 90 percent of the pandemic, indicates that less than one percent of adults have access to voluntary counseling and testing services and only about one of every ten pregnant women have the opportunity to benefit from intervention programs that can prevent maternal transmission of HIV.

Seventh, we are not aware of any ongoing effort to meet the shortage of health and development workers in Africa through a feasible, immediate deployment of employed and motivated professionals in the West. The widely praised recent initiative by the World Health Organization to provide lifesaving medicines to 3 million people in developing countries by 2005 relies heavily on training or hiring new health workers in Africa.

Finally, the logistic challenge of providing lifesaving medicines to more than 4 million Africans that the UNAIDS and the World

Health Organization deem qualified for urgent care should not be underestimated. These logistic challenges include training the local workforce, providing basic infrastructure such as potable water and basic sanitation, assuring constant electricity supply and telecommunication utilities to enhance coordination of services, developing verifiable management and clinical accountability systems, and improving epidemiological surveillance and reporting techniques.

What are we proposing?

We are proposing an International Volunteer HIV/AIDS Service Corps for Africa that will rely on a motivated volunteer in the West who is likely to continue receiving regular salary and other remunerations while on assignment. This volunteer will be linked through an employer or professional association to an agency or organization on the ground in Africa that is providing specific services in a specific target community, country, or region. We believe that if the opportunity exists to link a motivated paid volunteer in the West with an effective organization on the ground, many individuals quietly watching the unfolding tragic saga of AIDS in Africa will come forward and volunteer to serve to the best of their abilities.

The Proposed AIDS Volunteer Workforce

We propose an International Volunteer HIV/AIDS Services Corps to work on the following lines:

(1) It will match the desires of volunteers with the needs of target communities, countries, and regions in Africa.

(2) It will target countries with high rates of HIV transmission and those with low rates with the overall aim of preventing new infections, providing clinical care and support for those already infected, and keeping infection rates as low as possible in areas where they are low now.

(3) It will provide multidisciplinary services in chosen target populations, reflecting the multi-sectoral impact of HIV/AIDS. We envisage teams of volunteer doctors, nurses, public health experts, lawyers, engineers, economists, project managers, telecommunication

specialists, logistic experts and other professionals working together with the local work force in Africa to meet the needs of chosen target populations.

(4) It will recruit, in the first instance, individuals and organizations most likely to volunteer for service in Africa. These targeted volunteers will include African immigrant professionals in the West, Africans in the Diaspora (African Americans in the United States, African citizens of Canada, the Caribbean, Latin America, and Europe), and Africanists (non Africans) that have worked or grown up in Africa. Recruiting efforts will eventually target all other stakeholders.

(5) It will eschew bureaucracy by relying on volunteers for regular employment or those who can afford maintenance expenses required for the duration of work in Africa. We envisage, in most instances, a three-way understanding between the volunteer, the employer based in the West, and the agency providing a specific service in a specific area of Africa.

(6) It will train local staff and volunteers during their period of service to ensure sustainability of programs at the end of the volunteering assignment.

(7) It will specify a defined period of service, most likely one or two years in the first instance.

Technical Areas of Immediate Benefit

Africa is facing tremendous challenges in addressing preventive, treatment and support needs of individuals at risk or living with HIV/AIDS. An international HIV/AIDS volunteer program should assist Africa to meet the following immediate needs:

(1) Providing health, education, and social welfare support to 12 million AIDS orphans in Africa. At this time, there is no organized national or regional effort to address the needs of AIDS orphans in Africa. A multi-sectoral volunteer team of health workers, educators, social workers, and management experts can assist a specific African country to meet the needs of its AIDS orphans.

(2) Implementing community-based information, education, and communication campaigns against HIV transmission. A volunteer

multi-sectoral group comprised of experts in health education and communication, journalism, consumer marketing, epidemiology, logistics, and monitoring and evaluation will work closely with local counterparts to implement HIV preventive programs.

(3) Providing clinical treatment to individuals qualified to receive antiretroviral drugs. A volunteer team of physicians and nurses with expertise in AIDS care can work with its host country counterparts to extend clinical services to more individuals living with HIV/AIDS.

(4) Designing and implementing micro-credit schemes for women. Poverty and unemployment are major factors in the rising incidence of HIV transmission among African women. Providing steady employment or nurturing the entrepreneurial spirits of women can provide incentives and options against trading sex for basic necessities of life or for feeding small children. A team of rural economists, bankers, program managers, and small-scale entrepreneurs could work with host nation counterparts to empower women, especially young widows or women who lost their husbands to AIDS.

(5) Revamping healthcare infrastructure. A volunteer team of engineers, architects, project managers, energy and telecommunication experts, and health workers could assist health authorities in host countries to revamp existing services.

The above listing is simply illustrative. Each African country has needs that should be matched with skill sets of the volunteers.

Practical Implementation Issues

The proposed three-way arrangement between volunteer, employer and the agency on the ground in Africa will likely require additional funding for travel expenses and higher insurance premiums. We believe that the World Bank and the African Development Bank, two institutions that finance multiple projects in Africa, including the health sector, could cover travel expenses and insurance premiums for the volunteers. Bilateral agencies with major projects on the ground may also finance such expenses if it would speed up the implementation of their projects. Bilateral agencies from the United States, Canada, Britain, Germany, and Scandinavian countries finance multiple projects in Africa.

In addition, other multilateral agencies such as the World Health Organization, the United Nations Development Program, and the International Labor Organization may also be interested in facilitating the logistics of the volunteer program. Deep-pocketed foundations may also play financial catalytic roles. The key is to link with bilateral, multilateral, and philanthropic organizations already active on the ground in host countries.

To facilitate faster implementation of the volunteer corps, we propose an initial pilot period of two years with enough scale to make a difference in Africa. We anticipate pilot efforts in four potential settings.

(1) Major multilateral agencies: The World Bank and the International Monetary Fund (IMF) have more than 2,000 African professionals who serve in various capacities in various regions of the world. The management of these two institutions, for example, may enter into agreement with Unique to provide support services (health, education, and social services) to AIDS orphans in Southern Africa. The leadership of the World Bank and IMF will request volunteers from their African staff for a period of one or two years to serve on specific assignments in specific areas of Southern Africa, and pick up the salary and emoluments of each volunteer during the period of service. Depending on need and the number of volunteers, African staff in the two institutions will know in advance when they will be relocating for their volunteer service. We anticipate that other multilateral institutions can replicate the same scenario with their African staff.

(2) Organizations that cater to the needs of African Diaspora professionals in the West: In the United States, you have the National Medical Association (NMA), which represents more than 25,000 African American and other minority physicians. For example, the NMA may reach an agreement with the World Health Organization to provide 300 internist volunteers to help scale up antiretroviral treatment programs in Zambia, a country where there is one physician for every 14,323 persons, according to the World Bank. The NMA will seek volunteers from its membership, perhaps negotiate with the employers of members volunteering for service, and link the volunteers with the World Health Organization for the specific assignment in a specific part of Zambia. The World Health

Organization may pick up the transportation costs. Other Diaspora oriented organizations include the National Bar Association (NBA), which represents over 20,000 lawyers, judges, educators, and law students. UNAIDS indicates that 50 percent of all countries in sub-Saharan Africa are yet to pass national legislation ending discrimination against individuals living with HIV/AIDS. NBA volunteers can work with their local counterparts to develop legislation against HIV/AIDS discrimination either in the work place or at community settings. Another major organization is the National Dental Association representing more than 10,000 dentists and hygienists who can provide oral care, a major concern of AIDS patients battling opportunistic diseases.

(3) Academic institutions: These institutions can send their faculty due for sabbaticals to Africa as volunteers. They can also send students seeking field experience in Africa. Doctoral students and post-doctoral fellows, especially those focusing on African issues, can also participate as volunteers while continuing their research activities. Universities with medical, nursing, engineering, social services, and law schools can form a composite team of experts to tackle multi-sectoral HIV/AIDS issues in specific areas and specific countries in Africa.

(4) Business organizations with operations in Africa: These business organizations, depending on their areas of expertise, may rotate their volunteering staff to complement the community-based social welfare activities of their field operations in Africa. Volunteers may assist in information, communication, and education campaigns against HIV transmission. They may also provide technical assistance to local jurisdictions and civil society in setting up accountability mechanisms and assist in training or retraining local staff on personnel and logistics management issues. These volunteers may also provide technical assistance on community-based micro-credit services for rural women and other forms of activities that could increase the earning potential of women, and possibly reduce the need to engage in high-risk behaviors to feed themselves and their children. UNAIDS regards the interruption of male-oriented sexual networking in Africa as critical to overall HIV/AIDS remedial efforts on the continent. The

key is to match recipient country needs in the fight against HIV/AIDS with that of available skill sets in the West.

Conclusion

The HIV/AIDS epidemic is unusual in its scope and magnitude. An effective response must also be imaginative, creative, and tailored to meet the needs of target populations. Africa in the next decade will likely lack the requisite local workforce needed to mount a comprehensive, multi-sectoral response against AIDS. We believe that an international paid volunteer AIDS services corps can enhance the capacity of hard-hit African nations to scale up their response in the short term and assist countries with current low HIV infection levels to keep it that way. Remedial efforts against HIV/AIDS in Africa must marshal the extraordinary compassion felt by all men and women of goodwill into a call for service.

28

HIV/AIDS IN AFRICA: POLITICAL, POLICY, PROGRAM, HEALTH AND LEGAL RESPONSES *

(April, 2005)

I thank the leadership of the American Bar Association (ABA), the Section on International Law and Practice and the organizers of this conference for convening a discussion on Health and International Trade Law. Since the establishment of the World Trade Organization (WTO), the issue of international trade laws and access to healthcare goods and services has become an important global concern, especially in developing regions of the World. The 2001 WTO conference in Doha, Qatar ended with a series of declarations on international trade, intellectual property rights, patents, public health emergencies and the role of national governments in protecting the health of their citizens.

My discussion will focus on how African governments deal with the political, policy, health and legal dimensions of the epidemic. Since other presenters have discussed the trade law issues critical to effective HIV/AIDS remedial efforts, I will not dwell extensively on the burgeoning role of the WTO on access to public health goods and services.

Political Response to HIV/AIDS

Regarding the political response to HIV/AIDS, every African government, in my view, is clearly aware of the harsh political realities of HIV/AIDS. These harsh political realities include the potential decimation of emerging middle class; the erosion of hard-won national economic gains; the potential restiveness in military high commands if popular officers contract HIV and do not have access to lifesaving medicines; the destructive effects of runaway infection on each country's bureaucracy; and the possible electoral repercussions if a central government is deemed insensitive to HIV/AIDS.

The 2004 South African elections in my view marked a watershed HIV/AIDS political moment in Africa. The ruling party, the African National Congress (ANC), and the highly favored Mbeki administration found themselves on the defensive regarding national policies on HIV/AIDS. The ruling government campaigned vigorously on its future AIDS policies rather than on current or past policies. It is no secret that the Mbeki administration is one of the most powerful and effective governments in Africa. Yet the government had to make sure that South Africans who still have great affection for the ANC did not perceive the government as indifferent to HIV/AIDS issues.

Another effective role of strong HIV/AIDS response is emerging in Uganda. Today, Uganda's President, Yoweri Museveni is almost an icon in the West because of his courageous and highly effective anti-HIV/AIDS credentials. Consequently, very few Western governments wish to be on record regarding concerns about the future political transition in Uganda in 2006. The political intentions of President Museveni after 20 years in power remain murky. The political temperature in Uganda is heating up regarding concerns about an orderly transition when President Museveni's constitutionally mandated two-term period in office ends in 2006. .

Policy Response

The policy response of African nations to HIV/AIDS is heavily influenced by multilateral and bilateral agencies that finance HIV/AIDS remedial efforts in the continent. UNAIDS is a player with great influence on how African nations develop HIV/AIDS policies. UNAIDS has the capacity to deploy a vast arsenal of technical resources to assist African nations. Other multilateral agencies such as the World Health Organization, the World Bank, UNICEF and the United Nations Development Program also have leverage over national HIV/AIDS policies by virtue of their vast financial and technical resources compared to resources available to recipient African nations.

Another feature of AIDS policies in Africa is the tight control over implementation issues by central governments. This command-and-control policy making machinery creates concerns regarding the participation of national and local stakeholders in the design, implementation, monitoring and evaluation of national HIV/AIDS policies in Africa. To what extent are national AIDS policies in Africa reflective of the knowledge, attitude and perceptions of Africans affected or infected by HIV? Do national AIDS priorities in African nations represent the felt need of target communities? These concerns remain potent despite elaborate "stakeholder forums" or "consultations" that are common in national AIDS policy making in Africa.

Additionally, it is still curious that African nations are yet to take advantage of the explicit provisions in the Doha Declaration that allow impoverished countries to declare public health emergencies and consequently seek quality lifesaving therapies at the cheapest possible price. HIV/AIDS is already a public health emergency in many Southern African countries, yet current national strategies favor labor intensive and time consuming negotiations with research pharmaceutical companies that manufacture anti-retroviral drugs.

Another major policy issue is the lack of a continent-wide, coordinated policy on HIV/AIDS remedial efforts. Today, in Africa, any organization (public, private or non government) can initiate the implementation of its own version of HIV/AIDS remedial efforts as long as it can deploy financial resources. Many African governments are too poor and lack intellectual depth to engage multilateral and bilateral doors in serious discussions regarding national HIV/AIDS priorities. With the exception of the government of South Africa, and possibly Nigeria, it would be difficult to name other African countries with significant HIV/AIDS prevalence or incidence that have the clout to bend donor intentions to fit national HIV/AIDS policies.

Program Response

Lack of money and trained manpower is a major drawback to effective HIV/AIDS programming in Africa. Basic healthcare infrastructure remains a challenge. Limited logistical capacities represent additional impediments in Africa. For example, lack of potable water and basic sanitation in medical facilities or residential homes can have powerful influence on the ability of caregivers to provide quality care and support to individuals living with AIDS. Limited electricity supply can scuttle the best laid down supply chain strategy for delivering anti-retroviral drugs. Despite these concerns, the gravest challenge to HIV/AIDS in Africa is also difficult to understand.

The gravest challenge to HIV/AIDS programming in Africa, in my view, is the extraordinary disconnect between the frenzy of international HIV/AIDS remedial initiatives and the needs of individuals and families infected or affected by HIV/AIDS in Africa.

Today in Africa, a typical family battling HIV/AIDS is unlikely to receive any support or assistance from current national or international HIV/AIDS remedial programs in Africa despite high decibel media pronouncements. Less than two percent of individuals clinically qualified to receive anti-retroviral therapy in Africa receive these medications.

Another HIV/AIDS programming shortfall is the continued operationalization of remedial efforts as a health sector issue. The concept of a multi-sectoral response to HIV/AIDS is yet to materialize in many parts of Africa although the multidimensional implications of the epidemic are not in question. The lack of capacity to scale up successful HIV/AIDS programs in Africa represents another significant impediment. National governments in Africa continue to struggle financially and technically to support viable community-based HIV/AIDS programs. Non-government community organizations and secular organizations active in rural parts of Africa often have difficulties attracting sustainable national or international support for HIV/AIDS remedial programs.

In addition, African countries battling HIV/AIDS, to the best of my knowledge, are yet to mobilize their nationals living in the West to join the fight against HIV/AIDS. Countries with alarming physician-to-population ratios such as Ethiopia, Malawi, Zambia and Kenya cannot afford to ignore the potential role of their citizens working as health professionals in the West. Countries such as Nigeria, South Africa and Ghana with huge numbers of professionals living in the West have a ready resource that could play important roles in HIV/AIDS remedial efforts in their native countries.

Medical Response

Early stages of AIDS are often spent in hospital wards in Africa. As the condition worsens, most individuals living with AIDS go home to die. Hospital services in many Southern Africa nations remain over-burdened by the huge influx of individuals living with AIDS. The rising co-infection with tuberculosis among individuals living with HIV/AIDS is putting additional pressure on Africa's health systems. Lack of access to anti-retroviral drugs by individuals living with HIV/AIDS is effectively turning hospitals in Africa into mere "consulting clinics" where patients do not benefit from the expertise and knowledge of available medical expertise.

Another critical issue is the state of healthcare infrastructure in Africa. Healthcare infrastructures in many parts of Africa require urgent repairs or expansion to accommodate growing need. Financial support for these infrastructure improvements are often beyond the capacity of African governments. Unfortunately, infrastructure support is not always a priority of external donors.

In addition, the backbone of health systems in Africa, the community-based primary health care program, continues to deteriorate from lack of national and international support, exodus of trained staff and inability to maintain diagnostic and operational equipment. Community-based outreach programs with focus on information, education and communication campaigns also remain fragile as the budget for community health workers do not reflect unmet need.

Legal Response

The American Bar Association has an important role in assisting its counterparts in Africa to remove all vestiges of human rights violation and discrimination against individuals living with

HIV/AIDS. UNAIDS estimates that at least 50 percent of all African countries do not have laws protecting citizens living with HIV/AIDS from human rights violations or discrimination. In many African countries, the right to privacy of medical records is hardly enforced, and consequently, the idea of voluntary testing and counseling remains challenging.

Another critical issue is the need for legal reforms to end gender inequities in Africa. The inability of African women, especially widows, to own property in some parts of Africa, according to UNAIDS, is a major contributor to the growing rates of HIV among the female population. Widows with small children have minimal cultural rights to own property or inherit the joint savings accumulated with their late husbands. Legal sanctions against rape and sexual coercion need to be strengthened as part of comprehensive HIV/AIDS remedial efforts.

The American Bar Association can do specific things to assist individuals living with HIV/AIDS in Africa. First, the ABA can liaise with its counterparts in Africa to strengthen laws against human rights violation or discrimination against individuals living with HIV/AIDS. The ABA can send volunteers to work with national bar associations in Africa.

Second, the ABA leadership should encourage interested members to volunteer for short term technical assignments in specific African countries to meet specific legal needs. A major focus of this technical assistance could involve ABA volunteers and their African counterparts working closely with African parliaments in various countries to end human rights violation or discrimination against individuals living with HIV/AIDS. In another example, ABA members with expertise in human rights and trade law can provide technical assistance to African nations seeking to improve timely access to quality anti-retroviral drugs for their citizens.

These volunteer lawyers can also provide technical assistance to African nations engaged in negotiations with the often well-legally resourced pharmaceutical companies. They can also assist countries weighing their international legal options regarding generic drug manufacturing, drug re-importation issues, and declaration of public health emergencies.

Third, the ABA can organize training programs for its trade law colleagues in Africa and help link them, electronically, to top international and trade law libraries and databases. Interested junior lawyers can also volunteer to provide electronic legal research assistance to their African counterparts from their base in the United States.

Fourth, the American Bar Association can become a powerful advocacy voice for individuals living with HIV/AIDS in Africa. Today, barring unprecedented global and continental action in the next few years, the vast majority of more than 25 million Africans living with HIV/AIDS will die without access to available lifesaving, anti-retroviral therapy.

In the 21st century, millions of individuals may die of a manageable disease solely on the basis of geographical location, even when drugs that can prolong their lives are available. The ABA can play a powerful advocacy role with the US Congress and the White House to ensure that geography is not the ultimate predictor of highly avoidable deaths from AIDS. Today in the United States and Europe, HIV/AIDS is a chronic manageable disease and individuals living with the condition continue to be productive members of the society.

The ABA can also exert a powerful advocacy role in Africa by coming to the aid of individuals who are being persecuted because of their sexual orientation, political beliefs on AIDS remedial efforts or mobilization of target population for better access to health products and goods.

Fifth, the ABA can provide financial and technical assistance to non-government legal organizations in Africa active in HIV/AIDS remedial efforts. These organizations are active on human rights issues, gender inequity issues, representation of individuals living with HIV/AIDS in courts, and workplace discrimination against HIV/AIDS.

The key to an effective ABA role in international remedial efforts is the need to embrace the concept of a multi-sectoral response to HIV/AIDS. I have co-written a document on the need for an HIV/AIDS International Volunteer Services Corps in Africa with multi-sectoral technical teams from the West providing technical services to specific countries and on specific HIV/AIDS remedial issues (http://www.worldpress.org/Africa/2019.cfm). Depending on the specific needs of a country, ABA volunteers may work closely with their counterparts from the US-based National Medical Association, the Association of Scientists and Physicians of African Descent or other Western-based professional groups already providing volunteer services in Africa.

The intellectual depth of the ABA, the experience of its members in policy development, the fiscal reach of the organization and the deep pockets of some of its members could be deployed to effective use in international HIV/AIDS remedial efforts. The famed Pro Bono legal obligation for ABA members can be implemented in Africa as part of HIV/AIDS remedial efforts.

---

* Invited *Presentation at the American Bar Association, International Law, Spring Meeting in Washington, DC, April, 2005.*

29

RETHINKING THE GLOBAL WAR ON AIDS

(November, 2005)

The H.I.V./AIDS pandemic is now widely acknowledged as a major crisis of our time. As we gradually move to the third decade, the pandemic shows no sustained signs of slowing down, especially in hardest-hit parts of the world. It is crucial to step back and rethink current global remedial efforts.

According to the United Nations agency coordinating the fight against the pandemic (UNAIDS), almost 40 men, women and children worldwide live with H.I.V. Since the early 1980's, more than 20 million individuals have lost their lives to AIDS. Nearly 5 million people became infected in 2004 and 3.1 million died of AIDS during the same period. Sub-Saharan Africa continues to be the epicenter of the pandemic, accounting for more than 60 percent of all global infections although it represents only 10 percent of the global population. Southern Africa represents only 2 percent of the global population but accounts for 30 percent of all individuals living with H.I.V./AIDS. Nearly half of all adults living with H.I.V. are women. In sub-Saharan Africa, 57 percent of infected adults are women. The rate of H.I.V. transmission has also increased exponentially in other parts of the world in the last two years: nearly 50 percent in East Asia and 40 percent in Eastern Europe and Central Asia, respectively.

Despite these sobering statistics, the global war on AIDS includes clearly positive developments. It would be difficult to find a senior policy maker worldwide who has never heard of H.I.V./AIDS. Uganda's rate of H.I.V. fell from 13 percent in the early 1990's to 4.1 percent in 2003 through comprehensive prevention programs, according to UNAIDS. Spectacular advances in research led to the creation of life saving antiretroviral drugs that changed the pandemic from a deadly to a chronic and manageable condition in the West, with rates of AIDS death falling by up to two-thirds. The creation of the Global Fund to Fight AIDS, Tuberculosis and Malaria is a shining testament of global resolve to fight the pandemic. The unprecedented $15 billion, five year H.I.V./AIDS, TB and Malaria program of the United States in 15 developing countries represented another milestone in the scale and scope of a remedial effort.

Significant Obstacles to Remedial Efforts

However, in low and middle-income countries, extraordinary obstacles still loom. According to UNAIDS, although six million people qualified for life-saving antiretroviral treatment in December 2004, only 700,000 were on treatment. The commitment by the World Health Organization and UNAIDS to have three million people in the hardest hit countries to be on antiretroviral treatment by the end of 2005 has fallen short. The funding crisis for H.I.V./AIDS remedial efforts will soon reach crisis proportions as managers of the Global Fund scramble for money to meet future and current long-term commitments. I had addressed the looming H.I.V./AIDS funding crisis in another article on Worldpress.org.

In addition, significant obstacles impede access to preventive programs. Less than 20 percent of adults in hard-hit low- and middle-income countries, according to UNAIDS, have access to preventive programs. UNAIDS estimates that as much as two-thirds of all new H.I.V. infections in this decade could be prevented by expanding prevention programs to those in need. Fewer than 10 percent of pregnant women have the opportunity to receive services that can prevent maternal transmission of H.I.V. Less than 1 percent of adults aged 15 to 49 have access to voluntary counseling and testing services. No more than 3 percent of AIDS orphans receive any form of social support, especially in Africa. According to UNAIDS, by 2010, 18 million AIDS orphans will live in Africa.

What Is the Battle All About?

The bottom line is that new individuals become infected every day with H.I.V. Today, there is no known cure to H.I.V./AIDS. Every day, men, women and children die of AIDS. Every day, children graduate into the uncertain world of AIDS orphanhood. Every corner of the world is at risk. Some parts of the world are already waging a titanic life and death struggle with AIDS. Every day, about 13,423 individuals become infected with H.I.V. worldwide and approximately 8,493 die of AIDS.

It is critical to renew the fight against H.I.V./AIDS. We can build upon lessons learned in global remedial efforts. We can also modify or change ways of doing things as new challenges emerge so that individuals and families infected and affected by H.I.V./AIDS will have the best chance of survival.

What to do? I will briefly discuss possible changes in AIDS fighting strategies.

Proposed Changes in Global and Remedial Efforts

I propose that rethinking global H.I.V./AIDS remedial efforts should focus on the following issues:

1. End the ideological hard line battles over AIDS remedial efforts.

2. End all forms of means testing in AIDS programming.

3. End all obstacles to providing antiretroviral therapy to those in need.

4. Consolidate global H.I.V./AIDS remedial efforts in recipient countries into five areas of competency.

5. Deploy targeted resources for the training and retraining of health workers in AIDS-hit countries.

6. Governments of recipient countries should lead country-level remedial efforts.

7. Align poverty alleviation efforts with H.I.V./AIDS remedial programs.

8. Focus on community-based H.I.V./AIDS remedial efforts.

The foundation of a sustainable global response to H.I.V./AIDS is the availability of funds for the implementation of preventive, clinical and support programs. UNAIDS is now providing increasingly sophisticated and better-validated data on funding needs for global H.I.V./AIDS remedial efforts. The looming challenge is how to raise the $22 billion that UNAIDS estimates it would take to fight AIDS in 2007. In this regard, the United States has a special moral and fiduciary responsibility to ensure that enough financial resources are made available in the fight against AIDS. With strong U.S. leadership, other Group of 8 nations [Canada, France, Germany, Italy, Japan, Russia and the United Kingdom] will likely come through with additional resources. The pledge by Group of 8 nations during the 2005 summit in Scotland to fund fully H.I.V./AIDS programs worldwide by 2010 is commendable. However, the United States and other Group of 8 nations should ramp up their support to meet identified needs.

First, end the increasingly ideological and hard-edged battles over AIDS remedial efforts.

Today, international H.I.V./AIDS remedial efforts are over-shadowed by ideological battles between liberals and conservatives, between advocacy organizations and governments, between advocacy organizations and research pharmaceutical companies, and, between faith-based entities and secular organizations. Even Western countries face off from time to time, as shown during the 2004 International AIDS Conference in Bangkok when France accused the United States of attempting to force other nations to accept its strategic AIDS remedial policies. It is difficult to fathom how strident ideological battles can provide timely assistance to those in need. Anybody familiar with the suffering of families battling AIDS in Africa will fail to be persuaded on how ideological battles that delay or end remedial efforts can be useful to those in need.

All stakeholders in global H.I.V./AIDS remedial efforts should close ranks in the interest of the millions of individuals who die every year. I am not aware of any valid reason why closer cooperation and collaboration should not be the norm between generic and research pharmaceutical companies, between governments and advocacy organizations, between the private sector, governments and the civil society, and between Western nations and less-developed countries if the noble goal is to provide timely assistance to those in need. In this regard, the U.S. government has the capacity and influence to lead a global tone-down of the harsh ideological rhetoric on AIDS remedial efforts. No target population or individual at risk should be denied H.I.V./AIDS remedial assistance because of ideological differences.

Second, it is time to end any overt or covert means testing in H.I.V./AIDS preventive programs.

Since needless infections and subsequent deaths may occur with every day of delay, it is crucial for all stakeholders to embrace the ABC preventive approach (A for abstinence; B for being faithful to one uninfected partner; C for consistent condom use). No component of the ABC strategy should be given prominence over the other. In the war against H.I.V./AIDS, every proven method of deterrence must be utilized. As with all multiple strategic approaches, frontline workers and their managers who work directly with those at risk will have to customize their remedial efforts to meet the needs of their target population.

Rather than engage in battles over ABC, it would be better for AIDS planners, managers, researchers, advocates and funding organizations to focus on three key elements of behavioral change: the knowledge, attitude and perception (KAP) of risk taking and risk avoiding behaviors. In many developing countries, the KAP of the target population is rarely elicited, integrated or utilized in the implementation of H.I.V./AIDS remedial efforts. H.I.V. remedial efforts should also focus on how to empower at-risk populations to take charge of their health and avoid risk-taking behaviors that may lead to H.I.V. transmission. As noted by a group of prominent AIDS prevention researchers recently in the Lancet, a British medical journal, each and every individual ultimately has the responsibility for avoiding H.I.V. transmission.

Third, tackle all obstacles that impede access to antiretroviral drugs by individuals clinically qualified to receive these drugs.

According to UNAIDS estimates, six million people living with H.I.V./AIDS can begin receiving antiretroviral therapy, immediately. It is now accepted that access to lifesaving AIDS therapy is critical to expanding H.I.V. preventive programs. Consequently, any supporter of a comprehensive H.I.V. prevention program should also embrace the need for unimpeded access to antiretroviral therapy for those clinically qualified to receive these drugs.

There is a huge moral burden on governments, multinational corporations, financial titans, rich men and women, and major philanthropic organizations to determine why nearly 25 years after the emergence of H.I.V., individuals continue to die in the millions due to lack of access to readily available drugs. It is difficult to justify the current situation whereby living with H.I.V./AIDS and living in a developing country is a kiss of death.

To solve this moral hazard, it is important for three critical stakeholders to go beyond the call of duty:

A. Pharmaceutical executives worldwide, generic and research should come together and implement a Global Access to Antiretroviral Therapy Emergency Plan to make these medicines available to the six million individuals who will benefit, immediately.

B. Governments and multilateral agencies of the Group of 8 nations should provide adequate financial, technical and logistic support for the Global Access to Antiretroviral Therapy Emergency Plan. In particular, the U.S. State Department's Office of the Global AIDS Coordinator, which manages the $15 billion H.I.V./AIDS, TB and Malaria initiative, should work closely with both generic and research pharmaceutical companies to make lifesaving medicines available to those in need, and on time.

C. The Global Fund to Fight AIDS, Tuberculosis and Malaria deserves long-term support from Western governments and the private sector as a credible avenue for implementing multi-sectorial, country-originated H.I.V./AIDS programs and services in target populations.

To ensure the effectiveness of strategies that improve access to antiretroviral therapy, it is necessary to create a mechanism whereby available monies reach intended target populations in a timely fashion. The lag time between announcement of awards for AIDS programs and disbursement of funds is still troubling. The Global Fund, despite strategic, policy and operational priorities on program efficiencies and effectiveness, is occasionally slowed down by difficult negotiations with recipient countries or disputes over accountability issues. Global AID remedial efforts should minimize red tape. The ultimate solution is to devise innovative and simple accountability mechanisms that meet acceptable standards of financial and administrative probity in both donor and recipient countries.

Fourth, it is time to start consolidating global H.I.V./AIDS remedial efforts.

In the United States, as in other major donor nations, multiple agencies manage international AIDS programs. Most multilateral agencies have AIDS programs active in developing nations. International foundations and private sector organizations also manage AIDS programs in the developing world.

It is not possible to fight an effective global war against H.I.V./AIDS if bilateral and multilateral agencies, nongovernmental organizations and philanthropic foundations provide similar services and jockey for operational space in target countries. Perhaps during the incipient stages of the pandemic, it was necessary to elicit a response from multiple agencies and programs as scientists, health professionals and policy makers grappled with an unknown infectious disease. However, at this stage, it is difficult to justify even the remote possibility that H.I.V./AIDS remedial efforts may suffer from duplication of services or lack of coordination. In addition, resource-challenged countries battling H.I.V./AIDS should not bear the additional burden of managing the multiple demands, priorities and objectives of external donor-funded projects.

I suggest the consolidation of international AIDS programming into five core competencies, with bilateral and multilateral philanthropies and advocacy organizations eventually aligning their expertise and functions in target countries over a defined period. The consolidated core-competency approach to H.I.V./AIDS remedial efforts will ensure that the expertise of affected organizations become aligned with the needs and priorities of the target population. Every organization aligned to a specific area of competence will work together to coordinate their activities and share resources.

177

Today, most of the discussions on how to minimize duplication of services and potential wastage of scarce resources by external donors in recipient countries focus on country level coordinating mechanisms rather than the consolidation of service delivery. A consolidated H.I.V./AIDS remedial effort based on core-competencies will be beneficial as inherent economies of scale kick in when these organizations pool their financial and technical resources to tackle an identified need on the ground.

The five H.I.V./AIDS core competences include:

A. Research and evaluation (basic, clinical, quantitative and qualitative studies and vaccine development).

B. Strategy development, policy coordination and partnership issues.

C. Information, education and communication campaigns.

D. Clinical care and support.

E. Financing and logistics of care.

On research and evaluation, research institutions in donor and recipient countries are most likely to assume leadership roles. This consolidated approach will most likely accelerate ongoing efforts to implement genuine partnerships (twinning) between research institutions in the West and their counterparts in the developing world.

Regarding strategy development, policy coordination and partnership issues, UNAIDS is most likely to retain its current role as the technical lead strategic partner. In addition, UNAIDS' deep bench of policy guidelines and publications will serve as a guide on generic strategy or policy issues. However, deep-pocketed philanthropies such as the Gates Foundation will share a global partnership development role with UNAIDS since it currently finances some of the most ambitious global alliances against targeted diseases and health conditions.

For large-scale information, education and communication programs against H.I.V., bilateral agencies, foundations and advo-cacy organizations are likely to continue their leadership role as funding agents while host governments and community-based organizations in recipient countries lead implementation efforts at local levels.

On clinical care and support, the World Health Organization and medical institutions in both recipient and donor countries will continue to provide leadership, including long-term strategies for the training and retraining of local health staff.

A consolidated financial and technical core competency in recipient countries is most likely to be led by three entities with the huge economies of scale: The Global Fund, the World Bank and the Office of the United States Global AIDS Coordinator. The sheer size of the financial outlays of these organizations and their focus on eliminating financial and logistic hurdles to AIDS remedial efforts guarantees strong influence in this area.

In each recipient country, remedial efforts will also be organized around these five core competences to ensure seamless integration with external donor programs.

Fifth, training and deployment of health workers in Africa and other hard-hit regions is critical.

AIDS is messing up an already stretched health system in Africa. At least 95 percent of UNAIDS staff working in Africa in a 2004 survey indicated that lack of a qualified health workforce is a major hindrance in AIDS remedial efforts. Between 19 percent and 53 percent of deaths by government health workers in Africa is due to AIDS, according to UNAIDS. The health worker to population ratio in Africa is terrible: 1.4 health workers per 1000 people compared with 9.9 per 1000 in North America. This situation is made worse by the continuous migration of health workers from less-developed countries to the West. A revitalized international AIDS remedial effort should include a substantial outlay on the training and retraining of health workers in Africa and developed regions of the world. As of the time of this writing, I am not aware of a comprehensive, functional program to tackle the health worker crisis in Africa. In an earlier article in this section, my colleagues and I proposed an international volunteer H.I.V./AIDS services corps for Africa.

Sixth, government leaders in hard-hit countries should lead the fight against H.I.V./AIDS.

Two decades into this devastating pandemic, it is time to move beyond rhetorical and symbolic leadership on AIDS. Governments in Africa, the Caribbean, Asia and Eastern Europe should show long-term commitment by raising, substantially and permanently, the national budget on H.I.V./AIDS remedial efforts. In addition, national allocation to other healthcare programs should increase. Furthermore, no government in hard-hit countries should tolerate corruption and mismanagement of domestic and international funds. It is also crucial for governments of developing nations to seek ways of involving their nationals who live and work in the West in the fight against H.I.V./AIDS.

Seventh, align AIDS remedial efforts with poverty alleviation programs in hard hit countries.

Poverty remains a powerful inducement for high-risk personal behaviors that facilitate H.I.V. transmission. According to UNAIDS, poverty is at the center of the male dominated sexual networking in hard-hit countries that facilitate heterosexual transmission of H.I.V. Poverty alleviation programs should be aligned with AIDS remedial efforts at national and local levels.

This alignment must go beyond the poverty strategy papers favored by the World Bank and other development institutions. This alignment should focus on creating opportunities for wealth creation for low-income families. A key objective should be the implementation of female-friendly economic policies that promote entrepreneurship, property rights, human rights and wealth creation among women, especially young widows with small children.

Additionally, societal fault lines in hard-hit countries that could jeopardize hard-won gains in the fight against AIDS should be addressed. These fault lines include the role and status of women in the 21st century, enduring political and religious prosecutions of sections of the population, violent conflicts and wars over disputed lands and mineral resources, and damages to fragile ecosystems that destroy centuries-old means of livelihood. For example, in the

Democratic Republic of Congo, a successful H.I.V./AIDS remedial effort is unthinkable while the multi-country conflict persists and rape remains a prized bounty of war. A major AIDS initiative in the Niger Delta region of Nigeria, which produces the country's oil wealth, will require resolution of ongoing political, economic and environmental conflict between local inhabitants, oil companies and the central government.

Finally, shift the global war on AIDS to families and communities struggling to cope with the effects of the pandemic. The global war on H.I.V./AIDS should shift to villages, small towns, urban area and slums where families infected or affected by H.I.V./AIDS struggle to cope with the disease. To implement community-based AIDS strategies, it is important to develop measurable indicators for monitoring the impact of internationally funded programs.

As a start, I recommend that every H.I.V./AIDS remedial effort should respond to simple questions such as:

A. How many at-risk individuals changed their knowledge, attitude and perception regarding H.I.V. transmission, and ultimately changed their personal behavior through participation in specific international funded programs?

B. How many individuals clinically qualified to receive antiretroviral drugs receive them in a timely and consistent fashion through participation in specific internationally funded programs?

C. How many families infected or affected by H.I.V./AIDS receive support from specific internationally funded programs to meet non-health needs such as food, shelter, school fees, basic sanitation and so on?

Conclusion

The ultimate legacy of a successful global war on AIDS is how remedial efforts prevent new H.I.V. infection and how individuals living with H.I.V./AIDS receive timely clinical care and support services, including access to lifesaving antiretroviral drugs. Every year, millions of people contract H.I.V. Millions die of AIDS despite heightened global efforts. It is time to rethink current strategies. The war against H.I.V./AIDS is a race against time.

INDEX

A

Abuja, 57, 65, 68, 74, 91
ACTs, 89
adult prevalence rate of
   HIV/AIDS in Africa, 27
Africa Debt Relief-HIV/AIDS
   Swap, 42
Africa Development Bank, 94
Africa Working Group, 29
Africa. Lessons, 67
African children, xv, 44, 45, 46,
   87, 121, 127
African Development Bank, 41,
   46, 58, 95, 159
African Diaspora, 160
African extended family system,
   128, 135
African leaders, xvii, xviii, 33, 34,
   35, 36, 37, 41, 43, 50, 51, 57, 58,
   59, 61, 62, 65, 66, 113, 129, 138,
   140, 144, 149
African Leaders, viii, 33
African National Congress, 81,
   164
African-African American
   cooperation, 59, 145
AFRICARE, 98
AIDS crisis in Africa, xv, 45, 69,
   127, 134, 138, 143, 144, 145
AIDS orphans, xv, xxiii, 28, 45,
   47, 49, 50, 51, 54, 64, 69, 108,
   114, 121, 128, 143, 151, 158,
   160, 172
AIDS pandemic, xv, 33, 39, 41,
   72, 74, 123, 128, 129, 130, 131,
   136, 138, 141, 171
AIDS remedial efforts in Africa,
   xxi, 38, 41, 42, 51, 67, 79, 98,

143, 145, 146, 147, 149, 150,
   156
Al Gore, 127
Allan Lang, 143
American Bar Association, xxiv,
   163, 167, 168, 169, 170
ANC, 81, 82, 164
antiretroviral therapy, 46, 47, 68,
   77, 78, 115, 119, 145, 147, 151,
   154, 173, 175, 176
antiretroviral treatment, xv, 114,
   160, 172
ART, xv, xix, xxi, 28, 114, 115,
   116, 118, 119

B

Bill and Melinda Gates
   Foundation, 53, 54
Botswana, xvi, 28, 31, 57, 62, 121,
   123, 147, 150

C

Caribbean, 27, 91, 102, 147, 154,
   158, 180
CFA, 98, 140, 143, 145
Chinua Akukwe, 32, 38, 47, 59,
   60, 109, 132, 141, 142, 152
chloroquine, 89
CHRC, 47, 49, 50
civil service in Africa, 29
Clinton Administration, 98
co-infective status between HIV
   and TB, 94
Congressional Black Caucus, 53,
   55, 98, 132, 144
Constituency for Africa, 79, 98,
   99, 140, 141, 143, 145

D

E

F

G

H

Ordering this book and other books by Adonis & Abbey Publishers

Wholesale inquiries (UK and Europe):
Gardners Books Ltd
+44 1323 521777: email: custcare@gardners.com

Wholesale inquiries (US and Canada):
Ingram Book Company (ordering)
+1 800 937 8000 website: www.ingrambookgroup.com

Online Retail Distribution:
All leading online retail outlets including www.amazon.co.uk
, www.amazon.com
www.barnesandnoble.com, www.blackwell.com

Shop Retail:
Ask any good bookshop or contact our office:
www.adonis-abbey.com

+44 (0) 20 7793 8893

www.ingramcontent.com/pod-product-compliance
Lightning Source LLC
Chambersburg PA
CBHW020612270326
41927CB00005B/298